TECHNICAL
REPORT

A Review of Current State-Level Adverse Medical Event Reporting Practices

Toward National Standards

Megan K. Beckett, Donna Fossum,
Connie S. Moreno, Jolene Galegher,
Richard S. Marken

Prepared for the Agency for Healthcare Research and Quality

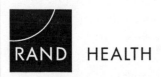

RAND HEALTH

The research described in this report was sponsored by the Agency for Healthcare Research and Quality (AHRQ) under contract number HHSP233200400145U. The research was conducted in RAND Health, a division of the RAND Corporation.

Library of Congress Cataloging-in-Publication Data

A review of current state-level adverse medical event reporting practices : toward national standards / Megan K. Beckett ... [et al.].
   p. cm.
   "TR-383."
   Includes bibliographical references.
   ISBN-13: 978-0-8330-3991-0 (pbk. : alk. paper)
   1. Medical errors—Reporting—United States—States. 2. Medical errors—Reporting—Standards—United States. 3. Medical errors—Code words. 4. Medical errors—Code numbers. I. Beckett, Megan.
   [DNLM: 1. Medical Errors—standards—United States. 2. Benchmarking—standards—United States. 3. Medical Records Systems, Computerized—standards—United States. 4. Patients—United States. 5. Safety Management—standards—United States. 6. State Health Planning and Development Agencies—standards—United States. WX 153 R454 2006]

R729.8.R48 2006
610—dc22

                                                 2006022126

The RAND Corporation is a nonprofit research organization providing objective analysis and effective solutions that address the challenges facing the public and private sectors around the world. RAND's publications do not necessarily reflect the opinions of its research clients and sponsors.

RAND® is a registered trademark.

A profile of RAND Health, abstracts of its publications, and ordering information can be found on the RAND Health home page at www.rand.org/health.

© Copyright 2006 RAND Corporation

Published 2006 by the RAND Corporation
1776 Main Street, P.O. Box 2138, Santa Monica, CA 90407-2138
1200 South Hayes Street, Arlington, VA 22202-5050
4570 Fifth Avenue, Suite 600, Pittsburgh, PA 15213
RAND URL: http://www.rand.org/
To order RAND documents or to obtain additional information, contact
Distribution Services: Telephone: (310) 451-7002;
Fax: (310) 451-6915; Email: order@rand.org

PREFACE

The Agency for Healthcare Research and Quality (AHRQ), an agency within the U.S. Department of Health and Human Services, is leading the national Patient Safety Initiative to combat medical errors and improve patient safety. As part of this initiative, states are encouraged to establish systems that require hospitals and other healthcare organizations to report information about the incidence, characteristics, and circumstances of adverse medical events. Ultimately, AHRQ would like to facilitate the creation of a national patient safety repository that aggregates data from states and other entities, such as hospitals and other healthcare organizations. This repository would enable analysts, healthcare organizations, and health policymakers to compare patterns of events across institutions—to determine, for instance, which adverse events are rare, which are frequent, and what circumstances are associated with the occurrence of particular events. Standardization of event reporting would also permit analysts to identify trends in adverse events over time.

This report summarizes the results of a 50-state survey of adverse reporting systems conducted in 2004 to document areas of commonality and identify variations in state reporting systems. The report also examines existing standards for coding health information in electronic databases, identifies issues that AHRQ will need to address in setting up a national patient safety repository, and presents an action plan to implement a standardized system for reporting data concerning adverse medical events nationwide. The action plan was elicited from an external advisory panel convened explicitly for this purpose. The analyses and observations presented here should be of interest to national and state policymakers, healthcare organizations, health researchers, and others with responsibility for ensuring that patients are not harmed by the healthcare they receive.

This work was sponsored by the Agency for Healthcare Research and Quality under contract number HHSP233200400145U, for which Robert Borotkanics served as project officer. The research was conducted in

RAND Health, a division of the RAND Corporation. A profile of RAND
Health, abstracts of its publications, and ordering information can be
found at www.rand.org/health.

CONTENTS

TABLES

SUMMARY

In 2000, the Institute of Medicine (IOM) published *To Err is Human*, which revealed that preventable adverse medical events resulting from human error pose a significant threat to patient safety and cost the healthcare industry millions of dollars. The federal government has a vested interest in improving the safety of healthcare. In keeping with the recommendations presented in *To Err Is Human,* the Agency for Healthcare Research and Quality (AHRQ) is leading the national Patient Safety Initiative to combat medical errors. One component of this initiative involves tracking change over time in the incidence of adverse medical events nationally. Currently, nearly half of states require or request that such events be reported.

A second IOM report, *Patient Safety: Achieving a New Standard of Care* (2004), recommended that efforts to achieve consistent standards for medical error reporting be undertaken. Standardized reporting systems can help to ensure that patient safety data are collected efficiently, used consistently, and shared appropriately across healthcare organizations and regulatory bodies. Used as intended, such systems can increase our understanding of adverse medical events and help us determine how to address them. To support these efforts, AHRQ contracted with RAND to examine several issues related to the design of adverse medical event systems. The research reported here aims to

- describe the adverse medical event reporting systems currently used by states and the accreditation bodies that evaluate healthcare organizations

- prepare a structured compilation of the data elements used in describing adverse events under these systems

- identify similarities and differences across state reporting systems

- determine whether existing methods of coding information regarding health and healthcare for storage and analysis in

electronic systems could be used to characterize adverse
medical events

- generate and organize ideas regarding the design and
implementation of a nationwide standardized adverse medical
events reporting system.

RAND SURVEY OF STATE AGENCIES

Between October and December 2004, we conducted phone surveys of
the agencies and departments responsible for hospital licensing and
regulation in each of the 50 states. During the phone interview, we
determined whether the state had a hospital reporting system for adverse
medical events. Our main goal was to identify systems that required
reporting of adverse events—singly or in the aggregate—that occur in
hospitals and other provider organizations, so long as hospitals were
among them. We collected detailed information about reporting systems,
including purpose, implementation date, type and format of information
collected, how information concerning adverse events is submitted to the
state, and what is considered a reportable adverse event.

To determine whether the goals of the systems we identified
reflected a concern with patient safety, we examined the system
documentation, looking for certain key words. For example, we
considered whether the legislation under which the system was enacted or
the description of the system developed by regulators used the words
"patient safety" or emphasized improving patient care rather than
punishing providers or hospitals for mistakes. We also requested all
supporting documentation, including codebooks, standard reporting forms,
and entity relationship diagrams, which are diagrams or flowcharts that
illustrate the structure of the information collected. In many cases,
our informants directed us to a Web site that contained much—but not
all—of the documentation we requested. In general, these Web sites
contained the law governing the system and the standard reporting forms.

With the documentation and other information provided by state
informants, we profiled each state system, using as a template to
organize our observations the IOM-recommended domains of patient safety
reporting. We created analytic files based on these profiles, which we

used to determine what types of information about adverse events states are collecting.

Results

Although we observed considerable variation across states in both the administrative procedures and the substantive aspects of the adverse medical event reporting systems we examined, the most striking result was the extent to which these systems had become more similar since the release of *To Err Is Human* (IOM 2000), a conclusion we reached by comparing the results we obtained with those obtained in prior surveys by the National Academy for State Health Policy (Flowers and Riley, 2000) and IOM (2000).

Administrative Characteristics of Adverse Reporting Systems. Our survey revealed that 24 states have at least one formal adverse medical event reporting system. Twenty of these systems are mandatory, that is, the healthcare organizations covered by the system are required to report certain adverse events to the state. General and acute care hospitals were cited most frequently as the kinds of facilities required to report adverse medical events, followed by ambulatory surgical centers, skilled nursing facilities, and psychiatric hospitals. Few of the states we surveyed were able to readily provide documentation about their electronically stored data (e.g., data dictionary, codebook, and entity relationship diagrams), and we found little agreement about what constitutes a data dictionary and codebook. The absence of formal documentation and definitions suggests a need for clarification and standardization to ensure that the adverse events reported to the system are categorized accurately, which is essential to cross-institutional or cross-jurisdictional comparisons and to efforts to identify trends in the incidence of adverse events.

Despite this lack of clarity, we were able to characterize the systems we identified in several important ways. First, nearly all of the systems we identified were oriented toward improving patient safety rather than disciplining misconduct. Second, although variations remain, states are moving toward the use of standardized methods of collecting and managing adverse event reports. For instance, most states require facilities to submit their reports using a statewide standard reporting form. Further, although most states currently permit multiple modes of submission (usually fax or mail), several states have adopted Web-based systems that demand more uniformity, and this approach appears to be growing. Regardless of how reports of adverse medical events are submitted, most states regularly store them in an electronic format of some sort, which, again, will facilitate comparative and longitudinal analyses. Only two states permit reporting of aggregate counts of events. The others all require reporting of each event defined as a reportable adverse event, another procedure that increases the feasibility of analyzing patient safety data to identify the frequency of various types of adverse events and the circumstances associated with them.

Finally, states are beginning to develop independent or semi-independent agencies to house the organizations concerned with collecting and managing patient safety data. For example, in Pennsylvania, the use of an independent agency has led to a very comprehensive patient safety reporting system. There are, however, some costs associated with this approach related to privity of contract concerns between the state and its vendors. For this investigation, these concerns meant that we were unable to obtain critical details regarding the system, including its data dictionary, codebook, and entity relationship diagrams. If it becomes apparent that systems housed in entities independent of the state are desirable for fiscal, procedural, or political reasons, it may be useful to determine whether there are ways to set up these systems that would permit analysts to have access to the data describing their components, configuration, and contents. Making this information available would help to promote transparency in efforts to monitor adverse events and would facilitate analyses of progress on patient safety concerns.

Procedures for Identifying and Describing Reportable Events. As with administrative procedures, our survey reveals increasing commonality across states in terms of the substantive information required by current adverse event reporting systems. Across systems, requirements concerning what events must be reported and what information about them must be included have converged. Even without a federal mandate to do so, most states have developed lists of reportable adverse medical events based fully or, more often, in part, on the 27 "never events" defined by the National Quality Forum (NQF),[1] the list of reviewable sentinel events identified by the Joint Commission on Accreditation of Healthcare Organizations (JCAHO), or a combination of the two. Since 2002, the number of states that require reporting of an NQF never event has increased for 23 of the 27 never events.

The most commonly included NQF never events are
- patient death or serious disability associated with a medication error
- wrong-site surgery
- infant discharge to wrong person
- wrong-patient surgery
- wrong-procedure surgery
- retention of a foreign object

The most commonly included JCAHO reviewable sentinel events are
- surgery performed on wrong patient or wrong body part
- hemolytic transfusion reaction
- rape.

The most common elements collected by state systems about reportable events are
- a narrative of the event
- information on corrective actions taken
- when the event occurred
- patient information.

---

[1] *Never events* are adverse medical events that, in a well-managed healthcare institution, should never occur.

ASSESSMENT OF THE UTILITY OF EXISTING MEDICAL STANDARDS FOR CODING ADVERSE MEDICAL EVENTS

A system for recording information regarding adverse medical events requires a coding system to capture information regarding the kind of event, where and when it occurred, who was involved, and so on. Thus, we set out to assess the extent to which existing standards for reporting health information in other contexts—that is, outside the context of patient safety—could be used to code the information in adverse medical event reports. More specifically, we attempted to determine whether existing health information standards could be applied to each of the IOM-recommended data elements for adverse medical event reporting.

We based our assessment on a review of the 27 standards identified by the Consolidated Health Informatics (CHI) initiative. Conducted under the leadership of the U.S. Office of Management and Budget, CHI is an effort to identify a portfolio of interoperability standards for health information. Our analysis suggests that efforts to develop standards for reporting adverse medical events can build on the CHI standards. Existing standards can be used to code much of the IOM-recommended information regarding adverse medical events. Many of the detailed standards already exist for particular data elements, such as patient and product information. Standards for other elements can be developed in the context of existing standards, such as the Systematized Nomenclature of Medicine (SNOMED) and the Logical Observation Identifier Names and Codes (LOINC), or through the efforts of such groups as HL7, which is a standards developing organization dedicated to providing a comprehensive framework (and related standards) for the exchange, integration, sharing, and retrieval of electronic health information.

Thus, it should not be necessary to develop special standards for coding information about adverse medical events. Such standards already exist or are being developed within the existing framework of other standardization efforts.

PROMULGATING NATIONAL PATIENT SAFETY STANDARDS

As part of our investigation, we convened an expert panel to discuss issues involved in developing and implementing a national adverse event reporting system. Panel members generally agreed that such a system should be simple, focused on adverse events that cause harm to patients (as opposed to capturing all medical errors), and administered by an organization that is not part of an entity that either provides or pays for healthcare. This last provision is important because, the panelists argued, ensuring the independence of a patient safety data collection and management organization would be essential to obtaining the cooperation of healthcare organizations and personnel.

A number of suggestions concerning the implementation of adverse medical event reporting systems were also offered. Perhaps the most important of these was that the skills of the people who would actually carry out the reporting need to be taken into account. Responsibility for reporting the details of adverse medical events is commonly assigned to healthcare personnel who have limited training, even though determining that a patient-harming adverse event has occurred may require interpreting complex medical data. To deal with this potential mismatch between task requirements and the skills of the relevant personnel, panelists suggested that, whenever possible, state adverse medical event reporting systems use predetermined menus to ensure that all of the essential details are reported using the correct terminology. Panelists also suggested that consideration be given to developing and using a set of "global triggers" that will automatically prompt healthcare personnel who are qualified to determine whether a serious adverse medical event occurred to review the relevant records.

The panelists also emphasized that employees must be assured that the information they provide will be handled confidentially and that the information will be used primarily to improve institutional practices.

Panelists noted, too, that rather than relying solely on incident reports to obtain information on adverse medical events, healthcare facilities should also audit patient records regularly to identify anomalous events, which can then be further investigated to determine whether a serious adverse medical event has indeed occurred.

RECOMMENDATIONS FOR ESTABLISHING A NATIONAL REPOSITORY OF PATIENT SAFETY INFORMATION

Our analysis of current adverse reporting systems, the existing procedures for coding information related to health and healthcare, and the views offered by our panelists lead to the recommendations below, which we believe will provide useful direction in the event that AHRQ moves to establish a national repository of state-provided standard patient safety information.

- **Create and maintain a database containing the information needed to track system characteristics over time.**
  Such a database should contain information concerning characteristics of the system, including the date it was implemented, when it was last modified, names of informants, their titles, and contact information.

- **Provide guidance to states regarding the supporting documentation for adverse event reporting systems.**
  To facilitate coordination and comparison across states, system characteristics and requirements must be documented. The federal government or another entity with experience in creating such documentation will likely need to provide guidance to states as to the types and formats of the materials needed and the format in which the data should be reported. In addition, as states move toward Web-based systems, additional guidance may be needed to develop database documentation that captures the characteristics of an electronic system.

- **In future research, determine how variations in definitions of reportable events affect cross-state comparisons of patient safety outcomes.**
  Many comparisons, and related validity studies, are needed to determine how particular variations in definitions of reportable events affect the assessment of patient safety outcomes. For example, researchers might compare adverse event rates under a system that requires that an event be reported only if it results in severe patient injury or death with the

rates under a system that requires the reporting of any
incident regardless of patient harm. Given the variety of ways
in which event definitions might differ, considerable research
will be needed to settle on a set of definitions that can be
used to reliable capture patient safety outcomes.

FINAL OBSERVATIONS

Although the *Patient Safety and Quality Improvement Act of 2005*
(Public Law 109-41) may increase the likelihood that states and
healthcare systems will focus on the development and implementation of
adverse medical event reporting systems, we believe that a national
adverse event reporting system with "teeth" will require federal
guidance. Even if mandatory state-level reporting systems are
implemented, it is unlikely that the states will achieve the level of
uniformity in their adverse medical event reporting systems required to
monitor the occurrence of such events nationally without such guidance.

The federal government could facilitate such a system by sponsoring
workshops to help the states develop a common set of standards for
tracking the safety of patients in healthcare facilities. The
government could also give grants to cover the costs of implementing
these standards. To reinforce the importance of maintaining these
systems, the federal government, in collaboration with the states, could
amend the Medicare claims processes to require that all healthcare
facilities receiving payments from CMS and having the agreed-upon
patient safety systems in place receive bonus payments. Concomitantly,
a dedicated unit within AHRQ could be established to assemble, analyze,
and report on the information provided to patient safety tracking
systems of all the states. This approach to standardizing the patient
safety tracking systems across the nation will undoubtedly take some
time to accomplish, but collaborating with the states in this effort
should help to ensure that all states buy into it.

There are two alternatives to a state-federal collaborative model.
The first—federal inaction and autonomous action by individual
states—will only produce newer versions of the varying outcomes
documented in this report. States will adopt and adapt guidelines being

promulgated by various entities, such as NQF and JCAHO, or they will adopt their own idiosyncratic list. There will be considerable variation in how information is collected, transmitted, and stored, thereby making it nearly impossible to develop a national repository of patient safety reports that could be used as a basis for monitoring progress and formulating policy.

The second alternative is direct federal intervention and control. This approach would require establishing yet another reporting system beyond those currently required by the states, the risk management systems implemented by individual institutions, and any other systems facilities may be required to participate in. In addition to imposing additional burdens on facilities (and thereby risking their support for such a system), direct federal intervention would be more costly and less efficient than collaborating with states. The results of our survey show that states have been quick to adopt or adapt reporting systems that incorporate recommendations made in *To Err Is Human* (IOM, 2000), suggesting that federal directives may not be necessary. It is possible, however, that states that have not yet modified their systems may be unwilling to do so in the absence of federal intervention.

ACKNOWLEDGMENTS

We want to thank people that we contacted in the state healthcare departments and other organizations who generously took time to discuss with us the adverse event reporting systems described in this report. We also appreciate their help in obtaining the documentation describing these systems that we needed to carry out our analyses. Without their help, we could not have completed this project. We thank the patient safety experts who, in their role as members of an external advisory panel, discussed with us their ideas regarding the form and content of patient safety systems, as well as issues associated with implementing such systems in healthcare organizations. The members of the panel were Anita Benson, Andrew Chang, J.D., Simon Cohn, M.D., Pamela K. Gavin, Lisa McGiffert, Harold Kaplan, M.D., Sanjaya Kumar, M.D., Lucian Leape, M.D., Arthur A. Levin, Jill Rosenthal, and Melissa Stegun.

We also appreciate the support and advice we received from Robert Borotkonics, our AHRQ project officer, and the many useful comments that we received from Michael Greenberg, Maureen Booth, and Peter Goldschmidt on an earlier draft of this report. Finally, we thank Donna Farley of RAND for her guidance throughout the project. Any errors of fact or interpretation are, of course, the responsibility of the authors.

ACRONYMS

ADE	Adverse drug event
AHRQ	Agency for Healthcare Research and Quality
ASA	American Society of Anesthesiologists
CDA	Clinical Document Architecture
CDER	Center for Drug Evaluation and Research
CDT	Current Dental Terminology
CHI	Consolidated Health Informatics
CMS	Centers for Medicare and Medicaid Services
CPT-4	Current Procedural Terminology
CVX	Clinical vaccine formulation
DICOM	Digital Imaging Communications in Medicine
DRG	Diagnosis Related Groups
EDS	Electronic Data Systems Corporation
EPA SRS	Environmental Protection Agency Substance Registry System
ER	Emergency room
FDA	Food and Drug Administration
GA-GDHR	Georgia Department of Human Resources
GA-PHA	Georgia Partnership for Health and Accountability
HCPCS	Healthcare Common Procedure Coding System
HHS	Health and Human Services
HIPAA	Health Insurance Portability and Accounting Act
HL7	Health Level Seven
ICD-9	International Classification of Diseases, 9th Revision
IOM	Institute of Medicine
JCAHO	Joint Commission on the Accreditation of Healthcare Organizations
LOINC	Logical Observation Identifier Names and Codes
NASHP	National Academy for State Health Policy

NDC   National Drug Codes

NCVHS   National Committee on Vital and Health Statistics

NDF-RT   National Drug File Reference Terminology

NQF   National Quality Forum

NYPORTS   New York Patient Occurrence and Tracking System

NCPS   National Center for Patient Safety

PA-PSRS   Pennsylvania Patient Safety Reporting System

PSA   Patient Safety Authority (Pennsylvania)

PSO   Patient safety organizations

RCA   Root cause analysis

SNOMED   Systematized Nomenclature of Medicine Clinical Terms

VHA   Veterans Health Affairs

1. INTRODUCTION

In 2000, the Institute of Medicine (IOM) published *To Err Is Human: Building a Safer Health System*, which brought the problem of medical errors to the attention of the healthcare community, as well as the general public, by showing that preventable adverse medical events resulting from human error pose a significant threat to patient safety and cost the healthcare industry over ten billion dollars annually. The issue has remained high on the nation's healthcare agenda. On July 29, 2005, after being passed by overwhelming majorities in both houses of Congress, the *Patient Safety and Quality Improvement Act of 2005* (Public Law [P.L.] 109-41) was signed into law by the president, thereby establishing a national system for the voluntary reporting of medical errors.

Under this law, hospitals and other healthcare providers will be encouraged to confidentially report information on medical errors to patient safety organizations (PSOs), entities that will be certified as meeting the criteria set forth in the law by the Secretary of Health and Human Services (HHS). The PSOs are to be placed on a publicly available list to be maintained by HHS. PSOs will analyze the information on medical errors that is reported to them and will give feedback to the healthcare providers about the possible causes of the medical errors that are reported, which will help to identify and implement possible ways to prevent those errors from happening again without fear of any of the supplied information becoming part of a lawsuit. The PSOs will then forward selected details about these medical errors to a network of databases, the creation of which will be facilitated by HHS, to give healthcare providers and others throughout the nation an "interactive evidence-based management resource" to use to conduct analyses as well as reduce medical errors and promote patient safety.

Early reactions to the new law, reported in the *Washington Post* (Gaul, 2005, p. A06), were mixed. One consumer advocate referred to it as "a teeny step forward." Jill Rosenthal, an analyst with the

National Academy for State Health Policy (NASHP), raised practical
questions about how the new law would affect healthcare organizations
in states that are already monitoring patient safety. In particular,
she noted that the existence of dual reporting systems could create
uncertainty about requirements for reporting to both the patient safety
organization and the state and about how the two reporting systems
might work together. Robert Wachter, a professor of medicine and chair
of the patient safety committee at the Medical Center of the University
of California, San Francisco, observed that the new law, although
symbolically important, would likely have little practical effect.
Apparently referring to the variation across the states on how adverse
medical events are currently defined and reported to state
systems—circumstances that the new law will not change, Wachter
described the present situation as "a chaotic mess" (Gaul, 2005, p.
A6).

One reason for the difficulties Wachter described is a
"disconnect" between the characteristics of traditional state-level
mandatory adverse event reporting systems and the key characteristics
of the patient safety reporting systems advocated in IOM (2000).
Traditional systems that predate the IOM report were designed to hold
hospitals accountable for the most serious mistakes made in the
provision of healthcare. Facilities were required to notify state
authorities whenever adverse events occurred—however adverse events
were defined. Generally, the state would then follow up to ensure that
some combination of on-site incident investigation and appropriate
institutional response occurred. In such systems, the state agency
could, potentially, impose fees and sanctions or suspend or revoke a
facility's license for failure to report such an event (Rosenthal et
al., 2001), but efforts to identify systemic problems that might give
rise to efforts to prevent similar problems in the future were rare.

In contrast, patient safety reporting systems of the sort described
in IOM (2000) are similar to risk management systems, which are
institutional activities that healthcare organizations—particularly
hospitals—undertake to prevent real or potential threats of financial
loss due to an accident, injury, or medical malpractice (Kraman and

Hamm, 1999). Risk management systems involve detailed assessments, including root cause analyses (RCAs), of adverse events. Modern patient safety reporting systems are similar to risk management systems in terms of what constitutes an adverse event and, in some states, in the requirements for detailed analyses of the circumstances surrounding the event. But the two kinds of systems have very different goals; whereas the purpose of risk management systems is to reduce human, facility, and financial risks associated with the operations of an institution, the objective of patient safety systems is generally to improve the overall quality of healthcare.

In keeping with the recommendations presented in IOM (2000), the Agency for Healthcare Research and Quality (AHRQ) is leading the national Patient Safety Initiative to combat medical errors and to improve patient safety. As part of this initiative, states are encouraged to set up reporting systems that require healthcare organizations to report to the states information that has traditionally been required only at the institutional level (through risk management systems). Examples of such information include RCA and risk assessment indices. Other key characteristics of patient safety reporting systems cited by patient safety experts include, in addition to confidentiality, are that they are voluntary (although some experts believe that reporting of the most serious adverse events should be mandatory), nonpunitive and undiscoverable in legal proceedings, timely and responsive, and easy to use (IOM, 2000; Cohen, 2000; Leape, 2002). In response, many states have sought to retrofit existing reporting systems so that they focus more explicitly on patient safety reporting. Other states that lacked reporting systems have recently implemented systems that are more similar to the patient safety systems recommended by IOM, while still other states have retained their original reporting systems.

In this report, we describe these diverse reporting systems. In particular, we focus on determining how the various state reporting systems differ in the kinds of information about adverse events included in event reports, a perspective that differentiates this analysis from previous studies of adverse event reporting systems. We focus on state-level adverse event reporting systems that cover hospitals, but, depending on the characteristics of the state system in question, also include other facilities (e.g., long-term care facilities).

The results of this analysis are intended to inform the development of a national patient safety repository that aggregates data from states and other disparate entities (Farley et al., 2005). In particular, the results in this report can be used to determine whether a core set of adverse events that states could incorporate into their systems should be established and, if so, what that core set of elements might be. We note that, presently, the federal government does not require states to adopt specific reporting standards, and we do not take a position on whether national standards should be adopted. But, even without national standards, institutional or state-level efforts to improve patient safety may profit from the experience of other institutions and states, and such cross-jurisdiction comparisons are most likely to be fruitful if they rely on similar reporting standards.

Standardization of adverse medical event reporting systems across states has potential benefits for state and federal policymakers, providers, and researchers. Access to a standard set of information about the occurrence of adverse events in other states would permit state policymakers to compare the performance of their own states with that of other states; for smaller states in which adverse medical events are rare, the availability of such a dataset would permit more statistically valid analyses of trends. For state and federal policymakers and researchers, standardization would enable a comparison of patterns of events across institutions to determine which adverse events are rare and which are frequent, and what circumstances are associated with the occurrence of particular events. Standardization of event reporting would also permit analysts to identify trends in adverse events across healthcare systems and to monitor improvements in patient safety associated with specific interventions, such as those implemented as part of the AHRQ Patient Safety Initiative.

The need for standardization is expressed in a number of NASHP[2] publications describing event-reporting activities under way at the state level (Flowers and Riley, 2000; Flowers and Riley, 2001; Riley, 2000; Rosenthal, Riley, and Booth, 2000; Rosenthal and Riley, 2001; Rosenthal et al., 2001). One theme running through these reports is the absence of federal guidance in the standardization of adverse event reporting systems, including definitions of adverse events and systems for categorizing—or coding—those events.

OVERVIEW OF THIS REPORT

As we have noted, state-level adverse medical event reporting systems, as they exist currently, vary from state to state and in the kind of information reported about events. In this report, we characterize the variations across states in the kinds of adverse events reported and in the information reported about those events; we also discuss the utility of existing healthcare standards for coding adverse event data. In addition, we conclude with an action plan to implement a standardized system for reporting data on adverse medical events nationwide. An external advisory panel that was convened explicitly for this purpose developed this action plan. In this section, we discuss these issues briefly and provide readers our main observations at a glance.

Which Events Are Reported?

Recent empirical work by NASHP (Flowers and Riley, 2001; Rosenthal et al., 2001; Rosenthal and Booth, 2003) found that, while more than 20 states had mandatory event-reporting systems that require hospitals and other healthcare facilities to monitor and report the occurrence of specific types of adverse events, the definition of a "reportable adverse event" differed across systems. Specifically, while all systems required the reporting of some types of unanticipated deaths, and most required reports of wrong-site surgery, there was greater

---

[2] See www.nashp.org (last accessed May 10, 2006).

variability as to what constitutes a reportable event beyond that. For example, Pennsylvania required the reporting of all hemolytic transfusion reactions, while Colorado required reporting of only life-threatening transfusion reactions (Rosenthal et al., 2001, p. 29-33).

Following an attempt to crosswalk the reporting requirements of 20 states with the National Quality Forum's (NQF's) list of Serious Reportable Events (NQF, 2002), Rosenthal and Booth (2003) documented the variation in types of events reported. The NQF list was used as a reference standard in the Rosenthal and Booth study because the original IOM (2000) report had urged Congress to designate NQF as the entity responsible for establishing and maintaining standards for a core set of reportable adverse events to be collected by states. NQF developed a list of clearly defined preventable adverse events that provided a benchmark against which to compare existing state requirements. The results of the comparison showed a high level of consistency in reportable events; it also illustrated the challenges involved in analyzing the overlap among event taxonomies (e.g., NQF's) and the diverse reporting categories used by individual states. The work of Rosenthal and Booth clearly demonstrated that, because of the heterogeneity in definitions of adverse events and ways of categorizing those events, the data gathered by the states did not provide an adequate empirical foundation for regional or national analyses of adverse events.

In Chapters 2 through 4, we discuss the methods and results of our survey of state agencies responsible for hospital licensing and regulation on their current state-level adverse event reporting systems. The results of this survey show that, in recent years, the tracking of adverse events is becoming more common, with greater consistency across states. Since the NASHP studies were completed, additional states have implemented adverse event reporting systems, and some states that already had such systems have overhauled them so that they are now more in line with IOM recommendations and event definitions generated by NQF and the Joint Commission on Accreditation of Healthcare Organizations (JCAHO). Most states that implemented adverse event reporting systems since 2001, the year that the NQF list of Serious Reportable Events was adopted, relied on the NQF list to develop their own event reporting requirements. We find that, despite the absence of any legal requirement to adopt a particular set of standards or the provision of federal resources to introduce new reporting systems, there has been a marked increase in the consistency of the types of adverse events that are reportable compared with prior surveys.

Because our survey focused on state agencies responsible for licensing and regulating hospitals, it does not take into account public health reporting systems pertaining to infectious diseases or other reporting systems that might measure hospital-based adverse events. In future work, we recommend that analysts try to capture other types of reporting systems that could help populate a national repository of patient safety outcomes.

What Information About Events Is Reported?

Medical event reporting systems differ not only in terms of how they define reportable events but also in terms of what information they request about these events. As noted above, this study differs from previous analyses of event reporting systems in that it not only identifies differences across the systems on which events are reported, it also focuses on the kind of information about each event included in individual event reports.

We refer to the different kinds of information that might be reported about an event as *data elements*. A data element is a specific kind of information about an event, such as the location where the event occurred or the likely cause of the event. Each data element can have different *values*. For example, possible values for the location of an event are the various locations within a hospital, such as the emergency room or critical care unit. The present analysis collected information about the data elements and the range of values used to describe the data elements in existing adverse event reporting systems. Our analysis, reported in Chapter 5, revealed considerable variation across reporting systems in the information (i.e., the data elements) required in reports of adverse events and in the values used to describe these data elements.

What is the Relationship Between Current Reporting Practices and Reporting Standards?

The IOM report on patient safety recommends a list of domains and related data elements that should be included in adverse event reports (IOM, 2004, p. 303). In this report, we use these recommendations as a basis against which to evaluate the consistency of the information included in various event-reporting systems; we use the NQF list of Serious Reportable Events as a basis for evaluating the consistency of definitions of reportable events. To evaluate the consistency of how the values of data elements are reported, we assess the extent to which current reporting systems conform to nationally recognized reporting standards.

In Chapter 6, we analyze the applicability of the HHS standards for health information data to adverse medical event reporting. We also compare the data element values collected by existing state reporting systems with the values found in existing American National Standards, such as X12N 837 (provider claims for payment); Health Level Seven (HL7) Versions 2 and 3; the Digital Imaging Communications in Medicine (DICOM) standard for imaging; and the national code sets and classifications for medical diagnosis and treatments and medical informatics standards adopted by HHS.

The results of these analyses indicate that developing a special standard for coding information regarding adverse events is unnecessary. The standards noted above, and others now in development, already provide systems for coding the information in adverse event reports. However, we find few data element values reported by existing standards. While existing standards can potentially be used to code adverse event reports, attention needs to be paid to standardizing the set of potential values that might be assigned to a given data element.

What Actions Should Be Undertaken to Promote Standardization?

In April 2005, RAND convened an external advisory panel composed of representatives of stakeholder groups, including providers of healthcare services, manufacturers of healthcare products, policymakers in the patient safety arena, researchers in patient safety and related fields, and consumer groups. The panel generated ideas for developing standard reporting requirements so that comparable information is obtained for a core set of events that can be compiled in a single system. The panel also addressed how this information might be shared (i.e., which standards-development efforts are promising). In Chapter 7, we summarize these ideas and, based on them, present a preliminary action plan for developing a core list of adverse medical events and elements about these events that states might incorporate into their systems to promote standardization of the reporting of adverse medical events.

In Chapter 8, we summarize the results of our analyses and present specific recommendations on how AHRQ and other agencies concerned with the development and implementation of adverse medical event reporting systems might proceed.

2. DATA COLLECTION AND ANALYTIC METHODS

OVERVIEW OF METHODS

In our investigation, we contacted state agencies that regulate hospitals to obtain information regarding their systems, if any, for collecting and storing data regarding adverse medical events. We requested copies of reporting forms, codebooks, and other documentation from these systems. Based on this information, we categorized states' reportable-event definitions and lists, risk assessment indices, and reports of causal analyses using a coding scheme that we developed. We recorded this information in a set of worksheets developed for this purpose.

SURVEY OF STATE AGENCIES

Between October and December 2004, we surveyed the agencies and departments responsible for hospital licensing and regulation in each of the 50 states. We first contacted the agency by email to explain the purpose of the study. We then followed up with a phone interview. During the phone interview, we determined whether the state had a hospital reporting system for adverse medical events. We used a broad definition of reporting systems so as to capture all relevant systems, whatever their content or form. Our main intent was to identify systems that require reporting of events, reported singly or in the aggregate, that occurred in hospitals. If the informant responded that the state did not have such a system, we asked whether there was pending legislation that might establish one.

If the state already had a reporting system, we undertook a semi-structured interview in which we asked for the following information:

- system name
- whether the system is mandatory or voluntary
- which facilities are required to report
- how a reportable event is defined
- the information requested about reportable events

- date the system was first implemented (or most recently updated)

- whether reports are made individually or in aggregate form

- what, if any, recoding of reported information is made after the information is reported to the state

- the name of the organization or agency responsible for administering the system

- contact information, name, and title for the person responsible for day-to-day maintenance of the system.

We also determined whether key words or phrases or concepts characterizing patient safety appeared in the legislation or in the documentation describing the state system. We searched for the phrase "patient safety" and searched for language that emphasized improving patient care rather than punishing providers or hospitals for mistakes. We suspected that reporting systems with such an orientation would be more likely to collect the type of information recommended by IOM and types of adverse events recommended by NQF and JCAHO. We also requested all supporting documentation, including codebooks, standard reporting forms, and entity relationship diagrams, which are diagrams or flowcharts that illustrate the structure of the information collected. In many cases, our informants directed us to a Web site that contained much—but not all—of the documentation we requested. In general, these Web sites contained the law governing the system and the standard reporting forms.

Few informants provided codebooks, data dictionaries, or entity relationship diagrams in response to our first contact with them. As a result, in April 2005, we contacted the states that had standard reporting forms a second time to request such supporting documentation. We restricted our second request for such documentation to those states because our initial interviews revealed that states without standard reporting forms were less likely to enter the information into a database or analytic file that could be used for a national patient safety database. Supporting documentation, such as codebooks, are relevant only when such analytic files or databases are maintained. In this second effort, we were more successful in obtaining supporting documentation that explains the data that are collected.

Nonetheless, we still found that the quality and level of detail of the information documenting adverse medical event reporting systems were uneven. In one case, the state was unable to produce the documentation in time for this report. And, after we had collected and analyzed our data, we learned that we had missed a system that had, in fact, existed at the time of our survey.[3] Our experience in collecting this information leads us to recommend that, for future surveys regarding adverse event reporting systems, researchers and research funders allow plenty of lead time for states to produce detailed documentation and to consider providing technical assistance to help states produce this documentation in a consistent and useful manner.

CREATING SUMMARY CLASSIFICATIONS

After we gathered information from the states about their reportable events and the type of information they collect about each event, we created a summary classification (see Table 2.1) of the specific vocabularies or classification systems used for reportable events and key characteristics to categorize the data elements that describe adverse events, such as risk assessment and causal analysis. Characterizing these vocabularies is an inexact science; in many cases, we had to rely on our best judgment. For example, we noted that several state reporting systems used the NQF short list of reportable events, with some modifications in the list's wording or additions or subtractions to the list. Other states based their lists on JCAHO

---

[3] When we initially inquired whether Maryland had an adverse medical events reporting system, we were told that it did not. We became aware of the Maryland system only after reading about it in a *Washington Post* article (Gaul, 2005). Although relatively new (it was implemented in March 2004, about six months before our research began), this system did exist when we collected our data.

sentinel events.[4] Still other states drew from NQF and JCAHO lists of adverse events or used their own "homegrown" event list that was consistent with state law. As described in Chapters 4 and 5, we used these existing classification systems and our own observations to create a summary classification system to categorize states' reportable-event definitions and lists, risk assessment indices, and reports of causal analyses.

Table 2.1. Classification Systems Used for Reportable Events, Risk Assessment Indices, and Root Causes

Data Elements	Classification Categories
Reportable events	• NQF's list of 27 Serious Events • New York Patient Occurrence and Tracking System (NYPORTS) • JCAHO Reviewable Sentinel Events • NQF 27 + JCAHO Reviewable Sentinel Events • Other List
Risk assessment indices	• USP MedMARx Error Outcome Categories • Veterans Health Administration (VHA) severity categories
Root-cause analysis schemes	• Eindhoven Classification Model (Battles et al., 1998) • VHA National Center for Patient Safety (NCPS) model (Bagian et al., 2001) • VHA NCPS + Eindhoven • Eindhoven (Medical) + JCAHO Reviewable Sentinel Events • Narrative provided by hospital staff

PROFILING STATE SYSTEMS

With the documentation and other information provided through the state survey, we profiled each state system. Our template was based on the IOM-recommended domains of patient safety reporting and their elements (see Table 2.2). We created analytic files (or worksheets)

---

[4] A *sentinel event* is defined as "an unexpected occurrence involving death or serious physical or psychological injury, or the risk thereof."

based on these profiles, as detailed in Appendix A. After all the information was added to the files, we emailed each of the states and asked them to verify all the information that we had for them; 15 of 22 states with reporting systems did so. The analytic files were used to produce the tables in Chapters 3 through 5.

Table 2.2. IOM-Recommended Domain Areas and Specific Elements for a Common Patient-Safety Reporting Format

The Discovery

   Who discovered or reported the event
   How the event was discovered

The Event Itself

   What happened, i.e., type of event
   Where in the care process the event occurred and/or was discovered
   When the event occurred
   Who was involved—functions, not names
   Why the event occurred—the most dominant cause based on a preliminary analysis
   Risk assessment: Severity of the event
   Risk assessment: Preventability of the event
   Risk assessment: Likelihood of recurrence of a similar event

Narrative

   Narrative of the event, including contributing factors

Ancillary Information

   Product information (blood, devices, drugs) if involved in the event
   Patient information

Causal Analysis[a]

   Technical, organizational, and human factors
   Recovery from near misses
   Corrective actions taken
   Patient outcome/functional status as a result of the corrective action
   Whether a similar case was recently investigated

Lessons Learned

   Safety lessons learned from the event

SOURCE: Adapted from IOM, 2004, Box 9-2.

[a]If a root cause analysis is carried out.

3. ADMINISTRATIVE CHARACTERISTICS OF ADVERSE EVENT REPORTING SYSTEMS

In this chapter, we summarize the number and general characteristics of the voluntary and mandatory adverse medical event reporting systems that we identified in our survey. We also compare, at a broad level, the results of this survey with the results of two previous surveys.

STATE REPORTING SYSTEMS: HOW MANY AND WHAT KIND?

Of all 50 states, the RAND 2004 survey done for this study identified 23 that have at least one formal adverse medical event reporting system. As shown in Table 3.1, of the 23 states that have such systems, 20 states have a single mandatory system and one state has a single voluntary system. Georgia reported having both a mandatory system—the Georgia Department of Human Resources (GA-GDHR) system—and a voluntary system—the Georgia Partnership for Health and Accountability (GA-PHA). As is discussed in Chapter 4, Georgia's mandatory system contains a subset of the larger list of reportable events in Georgia's voluntary system. New Jersey planned to implement a voluntary reporting system in 2006 (not shown in Table 3.1), in addition to its newly implemented mandatory system. When our data were collected, Oregon anticipated piloting a voluntary system in 2005. Finally, as noted in Chapter 2, we became aware of a 24th state, Maryland, with a mandatory reporting system shortly before completion of this report. Appendix B summarizes the information about each system that we obtained during the interviews.[5] A comparison of the RAND results with prior efforts reveals ambiguity and inconsistency in tallies of states with adverse medical event reporting systems over time. In 1999, IOM conducted a survey of all 50 states, and, in 2000, NASHP conducted a state survey. The results of the 2004 RAND survey, the 2000 NASHP survey, and the 1999 IOM survey are summarized in Table 3.1. Surprisingly, our 2004 results are more consistent with the 1999 survey and with the 2000 survey than the 1999 and 2000 surveys are with each other. Restricting our analysis to only mandatory reporting systems, the 2004 survey results

---

[5] Although not included in the body of this report, we do include a summary description of the Maryland system in Appendix B.

identified all of the 13 systems reported in 1999 and 14 of the 16 systems identified in the 2000 survey. However, the 2000 survey identified only nine of the 13 mandatory reporting systems reported in the 1999 survey. These discrepancies between the RAND results and the NASHP results are likely to be a consequence of the way that adverse event systems were defined; we describe these differences in detail in the footnotes to Table 3.1.

There is greater variability across the three surveys in the reporting of voluntary reporting systems than in the reporting of mandatory reporting systems. Specifically, in the 1999 IOM survey, no state reported a voluntary system. In the 2000 survey, five states (GA, NM, NC, OR, and WY)[6] reported having a voluntary system. In the 2004 RAND survey, New Mexico and North Carolina informants reported that they were unaware of a hospital-based adverse medical event reporting system. Oregon was piloting a voluntary reporting system in four hospitals and was still in the process of designing the system and determining what information it would collect.[7] Oregon had finalized its list of reportable events, however, so our discussion of Oregon's voluntary system is confined to Chapter 4, which compares definitions of reportable events across states.

The discrepancies noted in Table 3.1 illustrate the problem of launching new, independent surveys of state systems each time an analysis of adverse medical event reporting systems is conducted. Two factors may cause these discrepancies. First, variations in the definitions of what constitutes a reporting system can cause differences in what is included. Our definition of a hospital-based reporting system was broader than the one used in the NASHP study (see the table notes for Table 3.1). Although more inclusive in some ways, our analysis excluded Nebraska and Ohio, which NASHP includes. On the other hand, our survey captures California, Connecticut, Mississippi, and New Jersey, which the NASHP study did not. Second, gaps in informant knowledge—such as what occurred in our efforts to

---

[6] In our presentation of findings, we use U.S. Postal System abbreviations to refer to the states in parenthetical lists such as the one above or in tables such as Table 3.1.

[7] The state commission piloting the system expected that, by the end of June 2005, 50 percent of facilities would be reporting. We have no information as to whether this prediction turned out to be accurate.

determine whether Maryland had a state adverse medical event reporting system—may yield different outcomes in different surveys. Shortly after administering the 2000 survey, NASHP recognized and acknowledged problems of collecting data from state systems, many of which are the same problems we encountered, and corrected the information on their Web site and continuously updates the site[8].

The difficulties that NASHP and RAND encountered in developing a nationwide census of adverse medical event reporting systems indicate that informants in the state agencies responsible for hospital accreditation are not always aware of the presence of a state's reporting system.[9] Compiling information about and tracking state reporting systems would be more accurate and efficient if a database documenting system characteristics, as well as informants' names, titles, and contact information, were maintained by AHRQ or another entity that would be willing to share such information for subsequent data collection efforts.[10]

WHERE ARE THE SYSTEMS HOUSED?

Most adverse medical event reporting systems are operated by a state agency, typically the department of health, and sometimes a licensure or certification unit. In Minnesota, the state department of health assumed responsibility for the reporting system as of December 2004, but the state subcontracts much of the operation of the system to the Minnesota Association of Hospitals, which initially developed and operated the system.

---

[8]Maureen Booth, memoranda to authors, July 2005. The list of state mandatory reporting rules and statutes is available at http://www.nashp.org/_docdisp_page.cfm?LID=2A789909-5310-11D6-BCF000A0CC558925.

[9] It would be virtually impossible for a "false positive" to occur—that is, for an informant to report that an adverse medical event reporting system existed when, in fact, there is no such system— because informants must provide very detailed information to answer the survey questions.

[10] In seeking information for such a database, it is important that state officials be asked for permission to share their names and contact information with AHRQ.

Table 3.1. Results of Three 50-State Surveys of Adverse Event Reporting Systems

Survey	CA[d]	CO	CT	FL	GA	KS	ME	MA	MN	MS	NE	NV	NJ	NM	NY	NC	OH[g]	OR[h]	PA	RI	SC	SD	TN	TX	UT	WA	WY
RAND 2004[a]	M[c]	M	M	M	V/M	M	M	M	M	M		M	M		M			V	M	M	M	M	M	M	M	M	V
NASHP 2000[b]	M	M		M	V	M		M			M			V	M	V	V	V	M	M	M	M	M	M	M	M	V
IOM 1999	M	M	M	M	M	M		M		M			M		M		M		M	M	M	M	M	M	M	M	V

[a] RAND definition of a reporting system: A statewide adverse event reporting system that includes, but may or may not be restricted to, hospitals.

[b] NASHP includes only systems that are created through regulation or statute, are state-based, and relate to the medical management of a patient. Excluded are systems that require reporting of epidemic outbreaks, prevalence of communicable diseases, disappearance or loss of a patient, abuse, or neglect.

[c] M denotes a mandatory reporting system; V denotes a voluntary reporting system.

[d] We cannot definitively account for states with mandatory reporting systems that NAHSP missed but IOM and RAND included. Such discrepancies may be due to definitional differences in what is included or may be because NASHP's published report missed some states (that were subsequently identified and added to a continuously updated Web site). Because the Web site is continuously updated, we do not know which states that NASHP now reports as having a mandatory system should have been included in the 2000 report. However, we speculate that California and Mississippi may have been purposely excluded because they do not focus on medical management of a patient. New Jersey may have been excluded because it is created by "letter" rather than regulation or statute (as NASHP required). Connecticut may have been an erroneous omission.

[e] Maryland's reporting system was implemented in March 2004, but RAND did not learn of the system until this report was nearly complete.

[f] Nebraska's reporting system is based on reporting by facilities and professionals about actions taken against an individual licensed professional (such as revocation of the right to practice medicine or a malpractice judgment against the professional) rather than being based on reports of adverse events or incidents.

[g] In Ohio, facilities are required to report summary quality-of-care measures, such as length of stay, rather than adverse events or incidents, such as required by RAND.

[h] The system is not yet fully implemented.

Very recently, a few states have created adverse event reporting systems that are housed in independent or semi-independent entities. Of the nine states that report overhauling an existing system or implementing a new reporting system since 2003, three are housed in independent or semi-independent agencies. In 2003, the GA-PHA implemented the voluntary reporting system. In 2004, an independent agency of the Commonwealth of Pennsylvania, the Patient Safety Authority (PSA), implemented the Pennsylvania Patient Safety Reporting System (PA-PSRS). And Oregon's pilot voluntary system is being developed and operated by the Oregon Patient Safety Commission, a semi-independent state agency. None of the systems developed prior to 2003 are housed in independent or semi-independent state entities.

There are, potentially, both positive and negative implications of an increase in this type of organization with respect to the efforts being made to create a standardized national data warehouse of patient safety information. On the one hand, the PA-PSRS system is perhaps the most extensive reporting system in the United States. This comprehensive database could yield substantial amounts of information for each event, which could be desirable, assuming facilities are diligent about the information they provide. PA-PSRS personnel will also have substantial expertise and experience in analyzing patient safety information that could be shared nationally. Pennsylvania also had what appeared to be the most extensive and complete documentation of the system of any state. On the negative side, PSA, the authority responsible for implementing PA-PSRS was the only agency that was unable to provide us with critical details, including its data dictionary, codebook, and entity relationship diagrams, about the system because of the privity of contract considerations between PSA and its vendors.

Researchers and funders concerned with patient safety and adverse medical event reporting systems will need to be mindful of this issue, particularly if additional states follow the model of creating independent or semi-independent entities to oversee the reporting system. In future work, researchers will want to explore the pros and cons of the PA-PSRS partnership and determine whether the results of that analysis apply to all such systems. It would also be useful to determine whether there are ways to set up such systems that are housed by entities independent of the state that would permit analysts to have access to all of the data describing their components, configuration, and contents. If there are alternative ways of setting them up to facilitate obtaining such data, an organization such as AHRQ could develop guidelines for states that would enable them to create semi-independent agencies in such a way that data can be shared. This possibility assumes, of course, that the state's laws and regulations allow such information to be shared with federal and other entities. Because state systems have been set up to address state issues and may or may not have confidentiality provisions, states may not always be able or willing to contribute to a national repository of patient safety events.

WHICH HEALTHCARE FACILITIES ARE REQUIRED TO REPORT?

Table 3.2 shows which facilities are required to participate in all mandatory adverse medical event reporting systems. General and acute care hospitals were cited most frequently as the kinds of facilities required to report adverse medical events, followed by ambulatory surgical centers, skilled nursing facilities, and psychiatric hospitals. The "Other" category includes such entities as birthing centers, rehabilitation hospitals, and drug treatment centers.

One informant mentioned that there are problems with the level of detail that can be consistently reported when a range of facility types is covered by the same system. In this case, home health centers and other facilities that did not routinely deal with diagnosis and drug codes had difficulty using International Classification of Diseases, 9th Revision (ICD-9) diagnostic or other standard codes, so the state has moved away from requiring specific codes and is, instead, providing a menu or "picklist" of diagnoses and drug names.[11] Such issues may affect the feasibility of developing standardized codes that can be used reliably across different types of healthcare facilities.

---

[11] The term picklist refers to a drop-down menu of responses from which the reporter can select.

Table 3.2. Facilities Required to Report Adverse Medical Events in Mandatory Reporting Systems, by State

Facility Types	CA	CO	CT	FL[a]	GA	KS	ME	MA	MN	MS	NV	NJ[b]	NY	OR	PA	RI	SC	SD	TN	TX	UT	WA	WY
General/acute care hospitals	•	•	•	•	•	•	•	•	•	•	•	•	•	•	•	•	•	•	•	•	•	•	•
Primary care clinics	•										•												
Ambulatory surgical centers				•			•	•	•	•	•	•		•	•			•	•	•	•		•
Labs																			•				
Psychiatric hospitals	•						•			•	•									•	•		
Outpatient mental health centers	•																						
Home health centers	•									•		•							•				•
Pharmacies												•											
Skilled nursing facilities	•		•							•		•						•	•				•
Other	•	•				•				•	•	•			•	•			•	•		•	

[a] Skilled nursing facilities are not mentioned in the reporting instructions accompanying Florida's Code 15 reports, which describe in detail and analyze each serious patient injury, as defined by statute. The Florida informant added this category of healthcare setting.

[b] Starting in January 2005, New Jersey acute care hospitals were participating in a faxed-based system. The full Web-based system planned for 2006 will include all licensed facilities.

WHEN WERE REPORTING SYSTEMS IMPLEMENTED?

We asked states to provide information on when their reporting system was first implemented or, if the system had been modified since it was initially implemented, when the original system was updated or replaced. Table 3.3 shows the year of original implementation and, if applicable, the year the most recent system was updated.

DO STATE REPORTING SYSTEMS HAVE A PATIENT SAFETY ORIENTATION?

We reviewed the documentation that states provided to determine whether the system had a patient safety orientation. According to our definition, a system has a patient safety orientation if any of the materials provided to us describing the system used the term "patient safety" or if the documentation describing the intent or goal of the reporting system noted improvement of patient care or an emphasis on not punishing providers or hospitals for mistakes. Whether a system was judged as having a patient safety orientation is shown in Table 3.3, along with our findings regarding dates of implementation and updating.

We draw attention to two patterns. First, since the release of *To Err Is Human* (IOM, 2000), all reporting systems implemented or updated have a patient safety orientation. Second, of the 23 states having implemented a reporting system by 2004 according to the RAND survey, the documentation for the systems of 16 states is consistent with a patient safety orientation.

HOW IS INFORMATION ABOUT ADVERSE EVENTS SUBMITTED, STORED, AND DOCUMENTED?

This section describes the way in which states that have systems that were beyond the pilot phase as of early 2005 collect adverse event reports—that is, whether there is a standard reporting form that entities are required to use, whether healthcare facilities submit reports on single or aggregate incidents, how reports are submitted, and whether the information is stored in a computerized system. Table 3.4 summarizes these details.

- 23 -

Table 3.3. Year of Original Implementation, Year of Most Recent Update, and Patient Safety Orientation of Each System Observed in RAND Survey

State	Year of Original Implementation	Year of Most Recent System Update	Patient Safety Orientation
California	circa 1972	--	No
South Carolina	1976	--	No
South Dakota	1980	--	No
Massachusetts	1984	--	Yes
Florida	1985	--	Yes
Kansas	1986	--	Yes
New Jersey	1986	2005	Yes
New York	1986	1998	Yes
Colorado	1987	--	Yes
Mississippi	1993	--	No
Rhode Island[a]	1994	--	No
Washington[b]	1999	--	No
Wyoming	2000	--	Yes
Connecticut	2002	2004	Yes
Tennessee	2002	--	Yes
Georgia (GDHR/PHA)	2003	--	Yes
Maine	2004	--	Yes
Minnesota	2004	--	Yes
Pennsylvania	2004	--	Yes
Texas	2004	--	Yes
Utah	2004	--	Yes
Nevada	2005	--	Yes
Oregon	2005[c]	--	Yes

[a] Although its legislation does not have a patient safety orientation, Rhode Island expects that facilities—in having to report events, conduct peer review of incidents, and report corrective actions taken as a result of peer review—will find and implement ways to improve patient safety.

[b] Although Washington State legislation does not have a patient safety orientation, the Washington Department of Health is treating the system as if it has a quality improvement or patient safety intent and notes that the state does not object to this interpretation.

[c] Planned implementation date.

Table 3.4. Summary of How States Collect and Store Information

	CA	CO	CT	FL	GA-PHA	GA-GDHR	KS	ME	MA	MN	MS	NV	NJ	NY	PA	RI	SC	SD	TN	TX	UT	WA	WY
Aggregate reports	•						•													•			
Standard form		1	•	•	•	•		•	•	•		•	•	•	•				•	•	2		
Submission method																							
Telephone	•		•															•				•	
Telegraph	•																						
Fax		•	•	•		•	•	•	•		•	•	•					3		•	•	•	
Mail			•	•			•	•	•		•	•					•	3		•	•	•	•
E-mail								•										3		•	•		
Web					•					•				•	•				•				
Electronic																•							
Computerized system	•	4	•	•	•		•		•	•		•	•	•	•	5			•	•	•		

1 = Colorado requires use of a standard report for each of 16 reportable event types.

2 = Utah administrative rules state that the report shall be submitted in a Health Department-approved paper or electronic format. A Utah Department of Health Patient Safety Sentinel Event Reporting Form is available, but facilities have the option of attaching an internal form to avoid duplication of effort.

3 = Reports are submitted by phone, but they are followed up by mail, fax, or e-mail.

4 = Colorado saves submitted reports as PDF files.

5 = In 2001, the Rhode Island legislature funded a one-time effort to code information into an analytic file. Since then, no further funding for this effort has been approved.

Single or Aggregate Reports? Most states require facilities to submit a reporting form for each incident within a specified period following the incident or determination that an incident occurred. Two states (KS and TX) collect aggregate reports. Kansas and Texas require facilities to submit a tally of incidents by type, quarterly and annually, respectively. Kansas also collects reports on individual incidents that are determined by a facility's risk management department to fall below the threshold of standards of care, those with an injury occurring or with reasonably probable or possible grounds for disciplinary action by the appropriate licensing committee. This information is not tallied or entered into the state's computerized system.

Standard Forms. Most states' systems have a standard reporting form that facilities are required to use. Eight states (CA, MS, RI, SC, SD, UT, WA, and WY) do not use a statewide standard reporting form. With a standard reporting form, information can, depending on the mode of submission, be scanned or entered directly into an electronic format. A standard form also increases the consistency within a state about what event types and details about the event are both provided and can potentially be abstracted. In the absence of a standard form, information has to be abstracted from a narrative describing what happened. Utah, for instance, takes this approach. This difference has major implications for whether information can be collected and stored in a format that makes the data available for analysis—whether across time, across institutions, across event types, or for any other potentially informative breakdown.

Modes of Submission. Most states allow multiple modes of submission. The most common modes of submission are fax and mail. If the goal is to analyze incident reports to identify common problems, a Web-based submission method is ideal. As of 2005, five states (GA, MN, NY, PA, and TN) use a Web-based system exclusively. In Georgia, facilities that participate only in the mandatory GA-GDHR system can submit reports by fax. All reports submitted to the voluntary patient-safety system are submitted via the Web. New Jersey anticipates implementing a Web-based system in 2006.

We asked states with Web-based systems whether they had used a
vendor to develop and/or implement their system. Georgia and Tennessee
did not use vendors, although Tennessee originally contracted with a
person who was not, at the outset, a state employee but was later hired
by the state to manage the system. The Minnesota Hospital Association
developed Minnesota's Web-based system. New York used CGI-AM to develop
its system, and Pennsylvania is working with ECRI (with subcontracts
with the Electronic Data Systems Corporation and Institute for Safe
Medication Practices). Florida and New Jersey will select vendors to
develop their systems in 2005.

Electronic Storage of Reports. Fourteen states regularly store
information on adverse medical events in an electronic format. Colorado
stores the information in PDF files, which means that its data elements
are not easily analyzable. Rhode Island stores paper copies of the
reports; in 2001, its state legislature made a special request to
abstract this information for a one-time report on patient safety, but
this initial effort was not followed up. No additional funding was
appropriated for this activity, and no further reports were requested or
prepared.

Supporting System Documentation. We asked states that have
electronic files to provide us with documentation of the information
they have, requesting, specifically, data dictionaries, codebooks, and
entity relationship diagrams. Only Pennsylvania, which was unable to
share these specific documents with us because of the privity of
contract constraints described above, reported having all three sets of
documents.

Table 3.5 shows the supporting documentation provided by states
that collect standardized information and store information
electronically. States varied in the type of documentation that they
called "data dictionary," "codebook," and "entity relationship
diagrams." For example, Georgia PHA provided a data dictionary in the
form of a user guide, whereas Minnesota provided a data dictionary that
shows the list of variable names and labels. To facilitate development
of a federal database of standard patient safety reports from various
states, the federal government or other entity will need to provide

guidance to states as to what the various types of supporting documentation should contain and in what format that documentation should be, because any coordination across states will draw heavily upon such documentation.

Table 3.5. Supporting Documentation from States with Standardized Forms and Computerized Systems

Documentation	CT	FL	GA-PHA	ME	MA	MN	NV	NJ	NY	PA	TN
Data dictionary			•	•						1	4
Codebook		2	2			•				1	3
Entity Relationship Diagrams	•						•		4	1	•

1 = Information not released because of the privity of the contract between PA-PSRS and vendors.

2 = The codebook is reportedly Web-based, and the contact was not able to provide a hard or electronic version.

3 = In development.

4 = These materials were not available at the time this report was written.

We make two additional observations with respect to supporting documentation. First, as additional states move to Web-based systems, we expect that more complete documentation will become available and states can more easily compile analytic files to document trends and patterns. Second, in several instances, states did not have documentation on the systems that they could immediately share. Florida and Georgia each reported that their codebook is "Web-based" and that they could not print a copy. Tennessee was working to convert the documentation on its server to a format that could be readily transmitted and interpreted by RAND but was unable to accomplish this task prior to the deadline for this report.

STATES WITH PENDING LEGISLATION

If a state reported that it did not have a reporting system, we asked informants whether they were aware of any pending legislation that might establish such a system. Three states had legislation passed or pending that might result in an adverse event reporting system. In New

Hampshire, a House Bill (HB 518) to establish the New Hampshire Health Care Quality Assurance Commission was passed by the state House of Representatives and Senate in 2005. This legislation provides for the development of an adverse event reporting system. In Oklahoma, legislation to form a task force on patient safety was passed in 2004, but it was not certain when or if a mandatory adverse medical event reporting system would be established. In Delaware, a legislative initiative that would add a provision regarding the reporting of adverse medical events to the Delaware Code dealing with hospital regulations is pending. If the legislation were enacted, the issue of mandatory adverse medical event reporting in Delaware would be addressed in new regulations.

SUMMARY

Reflecting the variation in the history and objectives of state adverse medical event reporting systems, our survey of the 50 states revealed considerable variation in the ways in which states collect, submit, and store information about these events. Nonetheless, several states have taken the lead in establishing modern adverse medical event reporting systems by retrofitting systems that predate the patient safety movement or incorporating into recently implemented systems language and elements that are consistent with a patient safety approach. The focus on patient safety has been taken into account in some older systems and in all systems implemented or updated since 2000. There has been less progress in state-level procedures for collecting, submitting, and storing information in forms that will readily permit either analyses within states or cross-state comparisons. Taken together, these findings suggest that, while states may not need much direct guidance in incorporating patient safety issues into existing systems or creating new systems with language and intent consistent with concerns about patient safety, they may need guidance and/or resources in developing such systems to adapt existing systems to permit standardization in how information on adverse events is collected, submitted, and stored. These findings should be useful in subsequent efforts to develop recommendations for adverse medical event reporting systems.

An important limitation of our survey is that we contacted only hospital regulatory or licensing bodies. Thus, our survey did not identify any public health reporting systems pertaining to infectious diseases or any other reporting systems that might measure hospital-based adverse events. In future work, we recommend that researchers try to capture other types of reporting systems that could help populate a national repository of patient safety outcomes.

4. DEFINING REPORTABLE EVENTS

In this chapter, we provide an overview of definitions of adverse events used by the 24 hospital-based adverse medical event reporting systems surveyed by RAND for this project (See Table 3.1). We compare the definitions of reportable events to the NQF definitions of Serious Reportable Events and to the JCAHO definitions of sentinel events. We begin this chapter with a brief description of NQF and JCAHO event definitions.

NATIONAL QUALITY FORUM "NEVER EVENTS"

In *To Err is Human* (IOM, 2000), Congress was urged to designate NQF as the entity responsible for establishing and maintaining a core set of reporting standards to be used by the states. In response, NQF developed a list of six categories of "preventable adverse events," with a total of 27 specific events (National Quality Forum, 2002). The categories are

- surgical events
- product or device events
- patient protection events
- care management events
- environmental events
- criminal events.

Table 4.3 lists the full set of 27 preventable adverse events. These events, collectively, are called "never events," the idea being that they are events that, in a well-run healthcare organization, should never occur.

JCAHO SENTINEL EVENTS POLICY

JCAHO includes as part of its accreditation process a review of organizational responses to sentinel events. As noted in Chapter 2, *sentinel events* are unexpected occurrences involving death or serious physical or psychological injury, or the risk thereof. Serious injury specifically includes loss of limb or function. The phrase "or the risk thereof" includes any process variation for which a recurrence would carry a significant chance of a serious adverse outcome. Such events are called "sentinel" because they signal the need for immediate investigation and response.[12]

JCAHO-accredited organizations are expected to identify and respond appropriately to all sentinel events; an appropriate response includes conducting a credible RCA, implementing process improvements to reduce the risk of recurrence, and monitoring effectiveness of those improvements.[13] JCAHO makes available forms and instructions that organizations can use to respond appropriately to sentinel events, but organizations are free to follow their own internal processes. Organizations are also allowed latitude in defining "sentinel events," as long as they broadly adhere to the definition outlined above. A small set of "reviewable sentinel events" has been identified as particularly problematic and subject to review by JCAHO. Sentinel events are reviewable if

- the event has resulted in an unanticipated death or major permanent loss of function, not related to the natural course of the patient's illness or underlying condition, or
- the event is one of the following (even if the outcome was not death or major permanent loss of function unrelated to the natural course of the patient's illness or underlying condition):
  - suicide of anyindividual receiving care, treatment, or services in a staffedaround-the-clock caresetting or

---

[12] See http://www.jointcommission.org/JointCommission/Templates/GeneralInformat ion.aspx?NRMODE=Published&NRNODEGUID=%7bB37C3E00-728F-46AC-82AD-B6426A11ACCB%7d&NRORIGINALURL=%2fSentinelEvents%2fPolicyandProcedures%2f se_pp%2ehtm&NRCACHEHINT=Guest#one (last accessed July 13, 2006).

[13] Facilities can be accredited if, among other factors, the nature of health care practices is compatible with Joint Commission standards performance elements, JCAHO surveyors can communicate with all of management, clinical personnel, and about half of patients, and surveyors can understand facilities' medical records and documentation, and there is a focus on quality improvement (see http://www.jointcommission.org/HTBAC/HAP/hap_cah_eligibility.htm, last accessed July 11, 2006).

within 72 hours of discharge
- unanticipated death of a full-term infant
- abduction of any individual receiving care, treatment, or services
- rape
- hemolytic transfusion reaction involving administration of blood or blood products having major blood group incompatibilities
- surgery on the wrong individualor wrong body part.

HOW STATE SYSTEMS DEFINE REPORTABLE EVENTS

Table 4.1 presents a taxonomy that broadly summarizes how each state's adverse medical event reporting system has defined what types of events are reportable. There are three major patient safety frameworks: the NQF 27 Serious Adverse Events, JCAHO's sentinel events, and the New York Patient Occurrence and Tracking System (NYPORTS). Through conversations with informants or by carefully reviewing the wording of definitions of reportable events in the documentation, we found that states adopted one or a combination of two of these frameworks, or they created their own framework that reflected state needs at the time the system was implemented.

Systems in three states (CT, MN, and NJ) require facilities to report all or a subset of the NQF 27 serious adverse events. During our interview with, our New Jersey informant, the informant also indicated that the voluntary system being planned for implementation in 2007 would use an NQF list of near misses, if such a list were available. Our informant did not state what the alternative definition of near misses might be. We note that states generally vary the wording of reportable events to meet state law. For example, New Jersey modified wording of NQF events from reporting of "serious disability" to reporting of "harm." Future researchers will need to determine how these variations in wording affect the reporting of specific events. Such determinations are essential for reliable cross-state comparisons.

In the next two sections, we discuss in more detail how states *with* and *without* standard reporting forms classify reportable events. We conclude with a comparison of results produced by NASHP based on a 2002 update of state systems (Rosenthal and Booth 2003), and the results of the 2004 RAND survey on the number of all states (with and without standard reporting forms) with wording similar to the wording of the NQF serious adverse events and the number of states with wording similar the wording of each of JCAHO's sentinel events in 2004.

Table 4.1. Adverse Event Definitions Used by Each State's Reporting System

Approach to Defining Adverse Events	CA	CO	CT	FL²	GA-PHA	GA-GDHR	KS	ME	MA	MN	MS	NV	NJ^b	NY	OR	PA	RI	SC	SD	TN	TX	UT	WA	WY
NQF 27 Serious Events			•							•			•											
NYPORTS														•			•			•				
JCAHO Reviewable Sentinel Events						•		•				•									•	•	•	
NQF 27 + JCAHO Reviewable Sentinel Events					•										•									
Other List	•	•		•			•		•		•					•		•	•					•

New York instituted its first mandatory incident reporting system in 1986 and, in 1998, adopted NYPORTS, which is generally regarded as a leading state-based reporting system. NYPORTS was the first Web-based reporting system and is designed to provide immediate feedback to hospitals.[14]

Currently, the New York system has the following eight broad types of reportable incidents:

- patient deaths, injuries, or impairments due to circumstances other than those related to the natural course of illness, disease, or proper treatment

- fires or internal disasters

- equipment malfunction

- poisoning occurring within a facility

- patient elopements or kidnappings

- strikes by personnel

- disasters or other emergency situations

- unscheduled termination of services vital to safe operation of a facility.

NYPORTS provides a list of 54 "includes" events that fall within these broad event types. A very similar system—called the Unusual Incident Reporting System—has been implemented in Tennessee. Its taxonomy is like that of NYPORTS, but it uses different code numbers to indicate event types and has modified some of the event definitions. Rhode Island requires reporting of any of eight broad reportable events, seven of which correspond to the NYPORTS incidents listed above and 12 reportable incidents, ten of which are among NYPORTS "includes" events.

The reportable events specified in the systems of six states (GA-GDHR, ME, NV, TX, UT, and WA) are based on JCAHO's definition of sentinel adverse events and the list of reviewable sentinel events. States have shortened or—more commonly—lengthened the list. Georgia's

---

[14] See New York State Department of Health (2001) for a full description.

mandatory system requires reporting of only three of these events—unanticipated patient death, wrong-site/wrong-patient surgery, and rape. Nevada, on the other hand, lengthened the list of sentinel events by distinguishing among adult, child, and infant patient abductions and wrong discharges; it also added 12 events to the list (elopement, fall, homicide, maternal intrapartum, medication error, nosocomial infection, procedure complication, restraint, transfusion, treatment delay, treatment error, and a catchall "other" category). Texas added two events (patient death or serious disability due to medication error and patient death or serious disability due to use of device other than as intended), as did Washington (major failure or malfunction in facility and a fire that impacts patient care).

Two states—Georgia (GA-PHA) and Oregon—use a combination of NQF serious adverse events and JCAHO sentinel events. In addition to the three sentinel events that are required of the mandatory reporting system, the voluntary reporting system asks for reporting of events that fall within the six broad NQF categories (e.g., any surgical event) rather than the 27 specific events as part of its voluntary reporting system. Oregon's voluntary system will use a combination of NQF serious adverse events from each of six broad categories, with some (mostly semantic) variation in the definitions of these events and two JHACO reviewable sentinel events (unanticipated death or serious physical injury and infant death).

Ten states created their own lists or definitions of reportable events. While some of the items may resemble items included on JCAHO or NYPORTS lists, the overall reporting framework is homegrown. Kansas requires reporting of incidents that are found to fall below a minimum standard of care, with facility risk managers responsible for assigning final standard of care determinations and deciding which events are therefore reportable to the state. In the aggregate report forms, total counts of events that fall into each of the four levels of standards of care are reported.

REPORTABLE EVENT TYPES IN STATES WITH STANDARDIZED REPORT FORMS

The availability and use of standard report forms mean that facilities are reporting the same information about the same reportable events in the same way (and generally stored in the same format). Such standardization of information collected within a state will be essential to the development of a national network of reporting systems in which some of the information is captured and shared in a national adverse medical event data repository. Thirteen states, with 14 systems (13 mandatory, one voluntary) collectively, require the use of a single standard reporting form, and one state (CO) requires the use of a set of standard reporting forms with a different form for each reportable event.

To draw any comparisons across states about what events are reportable, we had to group these events into logical categories. To do this, we first grouped all events or definitions into one of the six NQF categories of serious adverse events. Within each of these six categories, we then further categorized events or definitions into a second and sometimes third level or hierarchy. For example, within surgical events, we identify six second-order groups (wrong site/patient/procedure, foreign object in patient/incorrect count, a combination of these two groups, death during or immediately following the procedure, complication following the procedure, and other). Third-order groupings were used to capture further distinctions among the categories of events. For example, within the wrong site/patient/procedure group, we identified four third-level groups: wrong site, wrong patient, wrong procedure, and combination of the above. We coded the events hierarchically and exclusively. This means that if a specific event is death due to wrong procedure, the second-order group would be wrong site/patient/procedure rather than death during or immediately following the procedure. We sought to classify first according to the type of error rather than according to the outcome because, in many systems, medical errors are defined by the incident rather than by the outcome.

There is a high level of consistency between the kinds of events reported in the 14 systems that have a standardized reporting form and the NQF list of 27 serious events and their six categories. (See Appendix C for a detailed presentation of the categorization of adverse medical events. Table C-2 is the basis for the following discussion of the event types in these 14 systems). Each of the 14 state adverse medical event reporting systems with standard report forms (including both Georgia's voluntary PHA and its mandatory GDHR systems) covers at least one care management event. Twelve systems include at least one type of surgical event and at least one patient-protection event, 11 systems include at least one criminal event, and ten systems include at least one product or device event and environmental event type each. At the broadest level, then, states are largely in agreement with NQF recommendations as to the types of reportable events that should be reported.

When we look at the second level of our categorization scheme (in Table C.2), which represents a slightly more detailed aggregation, we see somewhat less consistency with NQF events. Of the four surgical events on the NQF serious events list, six systems with standard reporting forms require reporting of events involving a foreign object left in a patient, and five systems with standard reporting forms require reporting of wrong-site, wrong-patient, and wrong-procedure events. At the third level of our categorization scheme, we see yet less consistency. Of the three product or device events, five systems with standard reporting forms ask for events involving a device being used or functioning other than as intended, and four systems each ask about contaminated drugs, devices, or biologics, or about intravascular air embolism. Note that, within these categories, there is variation in which events qualify. For example, four systems, as well as NQF, require reporting of an event involving contaminated products only if the event results in severe patient injury or death, whereas one state requires the reporting of any incident, regardless of patient harm.

There is greater consistency in the types of patient protection events between those systems with standardized reporting forms and NQF events. Eleven systems require reporting of events involving patient self-harm events, eight systems require reporting of an event involving patient elopement, and seven systems ask about events involving wrong discharge. With respect to care management events, nine systems ask about events related to medication errors (eight systems ask about the event only if the medication error results in serious patient injury), transfusion events, and events involving maternal complications. Four systems ask about adverse events involving hypoglycemia, hyperbilirubinemia, ulcers, and spinal manipulative therapy.

Of the environmental events, eight systems ask about falls (in seven systems, falls are reportable only if they involve death or other injury), seven systems require reporting of events involving burns and events involving restraints or bedrails, and four systems include reportable events involving electric shock or wrong or contaminated gases/substances. Finally, most systems consider criminal events to be reportable; such events include sexual assault (included in 11 systems), physical assault (eight systems), patient abduction (seven systems), and impersonation of a healthcare provider (four systems).

REPORTABLE EVENT TYPES IN STATES WITHOUT STANDARD REPORTING FORMS

Reportable events for states that do not require the use of a single standard reporting form are shown in Table 4.2. We reviewed the list of reportable events for each state and compared the way that these events that are reported with the language used in the NQF and JCAHO events definitions. We then grouped these lists of reportable events into the following three categories.

Systems That Emphasize Criminal Acts, Neglect, and Facility Failures

California, Mississippi, South Dakota, and Wyoming's lists of reportable events generally focus on events that are not usually associated with adverse medical events; instead, they focus on criminal acts (e.g., sexual abuse or rape), patient neglect (which tends to occur more frequently in long-term-care facilities), and infrastructure or service disruptions (e.g., fire or personnel strikes). Several of the NQF patient protection, environmental, and criminal events could reasonably be included in these lists, so if a standard form were created, reports could be combined into a national patient safety database. However, the reporting systems used in these states do not include all of the patient protection, environmental, or criminal events and likely none of the product or device events or care management events.

Systems Based on JCAHO Sentinel Events

Utah and Washington's list of reportable events are each based on the JCAHO list of sentinel events, with Washington adding two additional environmental events—facility malfunction and fire.

Other Adverse Medical Event Reporting Systems

As described earlier, Rhode Island's list of reportable events is based on a subset of NYPORTS items. The only reportable incident that corresponds directly to an NQF or JCAHO event is "Surgery on the wrong patient," although several other events are implicitly included. For example, Rhode Island requires reporting of events "subjecting a patient to a procedure/treatment not ordered or intended by the physician," which would capture wrong site and wrong procedure events. Rhode Island also requires reporting of serious complications that lead to extended stay or death, which should capture retention of a foreign object and death immediately following an ASA [American Society of Anesthesiologists] Class I procedure (i.e., a surgery involving a healthy patient, as classified by the ASA). Many of NQF's environmental events are likely to be considered reportable under the complication or malpractice report requirements. South Carolina requires reporting of incidents that result in death or serious injury and mentions, by way of example, medication errors and adverse drug events. While many NQF and JCAHO events would likely be included in this general definition, without the correct information, mapping the relationship between these events and the events specified in the NQF and JCAHO classification schemes would be very difficult.

Table 4.2. Reportable Events in States Without Standard Reporting Forms

State	Reportable Events
California	Occurrences such as epidemic outbreaks, poisonings, fires, major accidents, death from unnatural causes, or other catastrophes and unusual occurrences that threaten the welfare, safety, or health of patients, personnel, or visitors. Other occurrences include, but are not limited to, prevalence of communicable disease; infestation by parasites or vectors; disappearance or loss of a patient or inmate-patient; sexual acts involving patients who are minors, nonconsenting adults, or persons incapable of consent; physical assaults on inmate-patients, employees, or visitors; and all suspected criminal activity involving inmate-patients, employees, or visitors.
Mississippi	Suicide or attempted suicide, wrongful death, unexplained injuries, abuse, and interruptions of service at the facility.
Rhode Island	Reportable Events (1) fire or internal disaster in the facility that disrupts the provision of patient care services or causes harm to patients or personnel (2) poisoning involving patient(s) of the facility (3) infection outbreak (4) kidnapping (5) elopements from inpatient psychiatric units and elopements by minors who are inpatients (6) strikes, official strike notices, or other personnel actions that may disrupt services (7) disasters or other emergency situations external to the hospital environment that adversely affect facility operations (8) unscheduled termination of any healthcare service or utilities vital to the continued safe operation of the facility or to the health and safety of its patients and personnel. Restoration of utilities through use of emergency systems is not reportable.

State	Reportable Events
Rhode Island cont.	Reportable incidents (1) brain injury (2) mental impairment (3) paraplegia (4) quadriplegia (5) any paralysis (6) loss of use of limb or organ (7) serious unforeseen complication resulting in extended hospital stay (8) birth injury (9) impairment of sight or hearing (10) surgery on the wrong patient (11) subjecting a patient to a procedure not ordered or intended by the patient's attending physician, excluding procedures not requiring a physician's order, medication errors, and collection of specimen, for laboratory study, obtained by non-invasive means of routine phlebotomy (12) any other incident reported to the malpractice insurance carrier or self-insurance program.
South Carolina	Each accident and/or incident occurring in the facility, including medication errors and adverse drug reactions, shall be retained. Incidents resulting in death or serious injury (e.g., a broken limb) shall be reported, in writing, to the Division of Health Licensing within ten days of the occurrence.
South Dakota	Each facility shall report to the department within 48 hours of the event any death resulting from other than natural causes originating on facility property, such as accidents, abuse, negligence, or suicide; any missing patient or resident; and any allegation of abuse or neglect of any patient or resident by any person. Each facility shall also report to the department as soon as possible any fire with structural damage or where injury or death occurs; any partial or complete evacuation of the facility resulting from natural disaster; or any loss of utilities, such as electricity, natural gas, telephone, emergency generator, fire alarm, sprinklers, and other critical equipment necessary for operation of the facility, for more than 24 hours.

State	Reportable Events
Utah	Patient safety sentinel events include: (1) all deaths that occur at the facility and that are directly related to any clinical service or process provided to a patient for which the patient at the time of death (a) was not subject to a "do not resuscitate" order (b) was not in a critical care unit, except where the patient is transferred to a critical care unit as a consequence of a patient safety sentinel event that occurs elsewhere in the facility (c) was not in the emergency room or operating room having presented in the last 24 hours with a Glasgow score of 9 or lower. (2) events that occur in the facility and that are directly related to any clinical service or process provided to a patient and that result in (a) surgery on the wrong patient or wrong body part (b) suicide of a patient (c) major loss of physical or mental function not related to the natural course of the patient's illness or underlying condition. (3) events that occur in the facility and that are not directly related to clinical services provided to a patient and that result in an alleged (a) patient abduction (b) discharge of an infant to the wrong family (c) rape of a patient (d) intentional injury to a patient, whether by staff or others (e) suicide of a patient.

State	Reportable Events
Washington	(1) An unanticipated death or major permanent loss of function, not related to the natural course of a patient's illness or underlying condition (2) A patient suicide while the patient was under(3) An infant abduction or discharge to the wrong family (4) Sexual assault or rape of a patient or staff member while in the hospital (5) A hemolytic transfusion reaction involving administration of blood or blood products having major blood group incompatibilities (6) Surgery performed on the wrong patient or wrong body part (7) A failure or major malfunction of a facility system, such as heating, ventilation, fire alarm, fire sprinkler, electrical, electronic information management, or water supply, which affects any patient diagnosis, treatment, or care service within the facility (8) A fire that affects any patient diagnosis, treatment, or care area of the facility.
Wyoming	Allegations of abuse, neglect, misappropriation of resident/patient/client property; unexpected deaths; suicides; accidents with serious injuries; unexplained injuries or bruises; and infectious outbreaks. Medication errors that result in significant injury or death.

CONSISTENCY WITH NQF AND JCAHO DEFINITIONS OF REPORTABLE EVENTS

Our analysis indicates that there is some agreement across systems with standard report forms on the types of events that are considered to be reportable in state voluntary and mandatory systems. In this section, we consider the consistency of the state systems' lists of reportable events with NQF serious reportable events and JCAHO reviewable sentinel events. We updated a comparison done by Rosenthal and Booth (2003) of state and NQF definitions of reportable events and extended this analysis by comparing the language used in state-level definitions of adverse medical events with the JCAHO list of reviewable sentinel events.

Consistency with NQF

Table 4.3 shows that there are four events for which the number of states with event description language closely matching the NQF language did not increase from 2002 to 2004. Rosenthal and Booth (2003) report that in 2002 seven states use language closely resembling "surgery performed on the wrong body part," and six states use language closely resembling "surgery performed on the wrong patient," which is what we found in 2004. In truth, this apparent consistency between the findings for these two events across the two surveys is due to the fact that Rosenthal and Booth counted systems defining wrong-site surgical events as having the same or similar wording as wrong-patient surgery, and they counted wrong-patient surgical events as having the same or similar wording as wrong-site events. In the 2004 survey, we were stricter in categorizing systems as having the same or similar wording. We did not count wrong-site surgery as being the same or similar to wrong-patient surgery; neither did we categorize wrong-patient events as being same or similar to wrong-site surgical events. The other two events that remained the same from 2002 to 2004 in the number of states that reported the events the same way or similar to the way NQF describes the events were suicide (two states) and impersonation of a provider (one state). For all other NQF events, the number of states requiring that those events be reported has increased since 2002.

Table 4.3. Number of States in 2004 Requiring Same or Similar Event to
NQF, Compared to 2002

NQF Serious Reportable Event		Number of States with Language Closely Matching NQF	
		2002 (NASHP)	2004 (RAND)
Surgical Events			
1.A.	Surgery performed on the wrong body part	7	7
1.B.	Surgery performed on the wrong patient	6	6
1.C.	Wrong surgical procedure performed on a patient	1	6
1.D.	Retention of a foreign object in a patient after surgery or other procedure	4	6
1.E.	Intraoperative or immediately post-operative death in an ASA Class I patient	0	4
Product or Device Events			
2.A.	Patient death or serious disability associated with the use of contaminated drugs, devices, or biologics provided by the healthcare facility	0	3
2.B.	Patient death or serious disability associated with the use or function of a device in patient care in which the device is used or functions other than as intended	2	3
2.C.	Patient death or serious disability associated with intravascular air embolism that occurs while being cared for in a healthcare facility	0	3
Patient Protection Events			
3.A.	Infant discharged to the wrong person	5	7
3.B.	Patient death or serious disability associated with patient elopement for more than four hours	0	4
3.C.	Patient suicide, or attempted suicide resulting in serious disability, while being cared for in a healthcare facility	2	2
Care Management Events			
4.A.	Patient death or serious disability associated with a medication error	5	8
4.B.	Patient death or serious disability associated with a hemolytic reaction due to the administration of ABO-incompatible blood or blood products	0	4
4.C.	Maternal death or serious disability associated with labor or delivery in a low-risk pregnancy while being cared for in a healthcare facility	0	4
4.D.	Patient death or serious disability associated with hypoglycemia, the onset of which occurs while the patient is being cared for in a healthcare facility	0	3

NQF Serious Reportable Event		Number of States with Language Closely Matching NQF	
		2002 (NASHP)	2004 (RAND)
4.E.	Death or serious disability associated with failure to identify and treat hyperbilirubinemia in neonates	0	3
4.F.	Stage 3 or 4 pressure ulcers acquired after admission to a healthcare facility	0	3
4.G.	Patient death or serious disability due to spinal manipulative therapy	0	3
Environmental Events			
5.A.	Patient death or serious disability associated with an electric shock while being cared for in a healthcare facility	0	3
5.B.	Any incident in which a line designated for oxygen or other gas to be delivered to a patient contains wrong gas or is contaminated by toxic substances	0	3
5.C.	Patient death or serious disability associated with a burn incurred from any source while being cared for in a healthcare facility	0	3
5.D.	Patient death associated with a fall while being cared for in a healthcare facility	0	3
5.E.	Patient death or serious disability associated with the use of restraints or bedrails while being cared for in a healthcare facility	0	5
Criminal Events			
6.A.	Any instance of care ordered by or provided by someone impersonating a physician, nurse, pharmacist, or other licensed healthcare provider	1	1
6.B.	Abduction of a patient of any age	1	4
6.C.	Sexual assault on a patient within or on the grounds of a healthcare facility	2	4
6.D.	Death or significant injury of a patient or staff member resulting from a physical assault that occurs within or on the grounds of a healthcare facility	0	3

SOURCE: Adapted from Rosenthal and Booth (2003, Table 3).

Table 4.4. Number of States in 2004 Requiring Same or Similar Event to JCAHO

JCAHO Sentinel Event	No. of States with Language Closely Matching JCAHO
An unanticipated death or major permanent loss of function, not related to the natural course of a patient's illness or underlying condition	3
Surgery performed on the wrong patient or wrong body part	7
Suicide of a patient in a setting in which the patient receives around-the-clock care	3
Hemolytic transfusion reaction involving the administration of blood or blood products having major blood group incompatibilities	5
Unanticipated death of a full-term infant	2
Infant abduction or discharge to the wrong family	2
Rape	5

Consistency with JCAHO. Table 4.4 shows the number of states matching JCAHO sentinel events in 2004. The most commonly reported events with closely matching language are surgery performed on the wrong patient or the wrong body part (7 states) and hemolytic transfusion reaction and rape (5 states each).

SUMMARY

Even without a federal mandate to do so, most states have developed lists of reportable adverse medical events based fully or, more often, in part on the NQF 27 "never events," the JHACO list of reviewable sentinel events, or a combination of the two. In this chapter, we examined fully implemented reporting systems, both with (15 systems) and without (8 systems) standard reporting forms. Among systems with standard reporting forms, the number of states that use the same or similar wording increased for 23 of the 27 never events since 2002.

The most commonly included NQF never events are patient death or serious disability associated with a medication error, wrong-site surgery, and infant discharge to wrong person, wrong-patient surgery, wrong-procedure surgery, and retention of a foreign object following a surgical procedure. The most commonly included JCAHO reviewable sentinel events are surgery performed on wrong patient or wrong body part, hemolytic transfusion reaction, and rape. Among the states without standard reporting forms, two define reportable event types in ways that are largely consistent with JCAHO reviewable sentinel events. The definitions of reportable events in other states are likely to include NQF never events and JCAHO reviewable sentinel events, even if they are not explicitly based on those standards.

The definition of the kinds of events included in existing adverse event reporting systems provided here will, we believe, prove useful in efforts to achieve consensus on a list of adverse medical events types that states and organizations can use to measure patient safety processes and outcomes. In developing new systems or updating existing systems, the adverse events identified that appeared most frequently in our survey of current reporting systems might be regarded as the core of a new or updated system, with modifications or additions as needed to reflect the needs of the state and the kinds of healthcare organizations that will use the system.

5. DATA ELEMENTS: INFORMATION ABOUT REPORTABLE EVENTS COLLECTED BY STATES

To determine how states record information about adverse medical events, we analyzed the information collected by states about reportable events in terms of the data elements recommended in the IOM (2004) report on patient safety reporting standards. In this report, IOM recommended that health information systems be able to capture common data elements for the generation of multiple reports without redundant data entry. The data elements, shown in Table 2.1 in Chapter 2, represent the classes of information about patient safety events that IOM believes to be most important to the establishment of event reporting standards.

This analysis of data elements is based on data from 23 of the 24 state reporting systems identified in the RAND 2004 survey.[15] We reviewed the report forms and descriptions of required reports (if there was no required report form) for the 23 state reporting systems and categorized information requested on the forms in terms of the 18 IOM data elements listed in Table 2.1. Elements that did not fall into an IOM data element category were categorized as "Other Elements."

IOM-Recommended Data Elements Reported By Each State Reporting System. Table 5.1 shows which of the 18 data elements recommended by IOM (listed in the rows of the table) are currently included in each of the state reporting systems identified in the RAND 2004 survey (listed in the columns of the table).

---

[15] At the time of the interview, Oregon had identified what events were to be reported but had not yet finalized any other decisions regarding its program, including the information to be reported about an event. Therefore, the Oregon system is not included in the analysis of the data elements included in state reporting systems.

Table 5.1. Recommended IOM Elements Reported by Each State Reporting System

IOM Element	CA	CO	CT	FL	GA-PHA	GA-GDHR	KS	ME	MA	MN	MI	NV	NJ	NY	PA	RI	SC	SD	TN	TX	UT	WA	WY
Role of the person who discovered event	•	•																					
How event was discovered		•	•	•					•				•	•	•				•				
Where in the care process the event was discovered		•	•	•					•		•	•	•	•	•				•		•		
When the event occurred	•	•	•	•	•	•	•	•	•	•	•	•	•	•	•				•		•		
Function of those involved		•		•					•					•					•				
Most dominant cause based on preliminary analysis		•		•	•			•			•				•								
Risk assessment: Severity of event					•																		
Risk assessment: Preventability of event										•			•		•								
Risk assessment: Likelihood of recurrence															•								
Narrative of the event	•	•	•	•	•	•	•	•	•	•	•		•	•	•	•	•	•	•		•	•	•
Product information		•		•					•				•	•	•				•				
Patient information		•	•	•		•		•	•	•		•	•	•	•				•		•		
Causal analysis: Technical, organizations, and human factors					•					•		•	•	•	•				•		•		•
Causal analysis: Recovery from near misses																							
Causal analysis: Corrective actions taken		•	•	•	•	•	•	•	•	•	•	•	•	•	•	•			•	•	•		•
Causal analysis: Patient outcome/functional status		•											•	•	•	•			•				
Causal analysis: What a similar case recently investigated		•							•														
Lessons Learned							•					•		•	•								

The data element most often included in state reporting systems is a narrative description of the event. Twenty of the 23 reporting systems require such a description.

The next most prevalent data element is "Causal analysis: Corrective actions taken." Eighteen of the 23 state reporting systems require a description of corrective actions taken to prevent future occurrences of the event. More than half of the state reporting systems also require that healthcare organizations report "When event occurred" and "Patient information." Some of the information recommended by the IOM is not currently included in any reporting system. No reporting system currently collects information regarding the preventability of the event ("Risk assessment: preventability") or about recovery from near misses ("Causal analysis: Recovery from near misses").

Number of Data Elements Reported by Each State System. Of the possible 18 IOM-recommended data elements shown in Table 2.1 (with exception of event type), the largest number included in any state report is 13 (PA), and the smallest number is one (SC, SD, and WA). Only six of the 23 state reporting systems (CO, FL, MA, NJ, NY, PA, and TN) include at least half of these IOM-recommended data elements.

DATA ELEMENT DETAILS

In this section, we describe in some detail the cross-state variations in the kind of information requested for the different data elements.

DISCOVERY OF ADVERSE EVENTS

There are two data elements that pertain to the discovery of adverse events: the role of the person who discovered the event and how the event was discovered.

Role of Person Who Discovered the Event. Only one state system (CO) asks for the name of the person who discovered the event, but it does not ask for this information in terms of the title or position of the person who discovered the event, as recommended by the IOM. Nine other state systems ask only for the title or position of the person who filed the report—not the person who discovered the event. The person who filed the report may or may not be the person who discovered the event being reported. Therefore, we did not count these data elements as being consistent with the IOM recommendation that reports include information about the role of the person who actually discovered the event.

How the Event Was Discovered. Six state systems (CO, FL, MA, NJ, PA, and TN) request information regarding how the event was discovered. Two systems (NJ and PA) have a fixed list of options regarding how the event was discovered. The options include

- report by staff

- report by family/visitor

- report by patient

- assessment after event

- review of chart/record.

Two state systems (CO and TN) ask for a textual description of how the event was discovered; in Colorado, this description is only obtained for events involving missing medication. Four systems (CO, FL, MA, and PA) ask whether there was a witness to the event. If there was a witness, these states ask either for the name or license number of the witness.

THE EVENT ITSELF

In addition to type of event (discussed in Chapter 4), IOM recommended that medical event reporting systems supply the following seven elements of information regarding the event itself:

- where in the care process the event was discovered

- when the event occurred

- function of those involved

- most dominant cause based on preliminary analysis

- risk assessment: severity of the event

- risk assessment: preventability of the event

- risk assessment: likelihood of recurrence of a similar event.

Where in the Care Process the Event Was Discovered and/or Occurred.
Eleven state reporting systems (CO, CT, FL, MA, MS, NV, NJ, NY, PA, TN, and UT) request information about where in the care process the event was discovered and/or occurred. However, there is considerable variation across systems in terms of the options available for providing this information. To some extent, this variation may depend on the type of healthcare facilities that provide event reports to the state system. Table 5.2 shows the options available for reporting where in the care process an event occurred for each of the systems that requires such information.

Six of the systems shown in Table 5.2 (CO, CT, FL, NV, NJ, and NY) provide options for indicating the name of a hospital unit where the event occurred. These options always include the emergency room (ER) and intensive care unit (ICU). Four systems (MA, MS, PA, and UT) require only a text description of where in the care process the event occurred. Two systems (NJ and TN) require information about where in the medication process (prescribing, transcription, preparation, or administration) the event occurred when the event was a medication error.

Table 5.2. Options for Specifying Where in the Care Process an Event Was Discovered or Occurred

	CO	CT	FL	MA	MS	NV	NJ	NY	PA	TN	UT
Cardiac		•	•			•		•			
Dialysis		•				•		•			
ER	•	•	•			•	•	•			
ICU	•	•	•			•	•	•			
Laboratory			•			•	•	•			
Maternity		•	•			•	•	•			
Patient's room			•				•	•			
Pediatric		•				•					
Psychiatric	•	•				•					
Rehab	•	•	•				•	•			
Surgical		•	•			•	•	•			
Common area							•	•			

	CO	CT	FL	MA	MS	NV	NJ	NY	PA	TN	UT
Describe location (text)				•	•			•	•		•
Other hospital unit		•	•			•	•	•			
Assisted care			•								
Where in medication process (text)							•			•	
Outpatient		•	•			•		•			
Other provider			•								

When the Event Occurred. Seventeen state reporting systems (CA, CO, CT, FL, GA-PHA, GA-GDHR, KS, ME, MA, MN, MS, NV, NJ, NY, PA, TN, and UT) ask for information about when the event occurred. One system (NV) asks for information about when the report was filed. The information about when the event occurred that is included in different state reporting systems is summarized in Table 5.3. Most systems ask for both the time and date of the event. But some systems (CA and GA-GDHR) ask only for the time of the event, while others (KS, NV, and UT) ask only for the date of the event. Reporting systems also differ in terms of the required format of the information requested for the time and date of the event (MM/DD/YY vs. text entry, for example) (results not shown).

Table 5.3. Options for Specifying When the Event Occurred

When Event Occurred	CA	CO	CT	FL	GA-PHA	GA-GDHR	KS	ME	MA	MN	MS	NV	NJ	NY	PA	TN	UT
Event date		•	•	•	•	•	•	•	•	•	•	•	•	•	•	•	•
Time	•	•	•	•	•	•		•	•	•	•			•	•	•	
Date/Time of event		•												•			
Date/Time of report												•					

Function of Those Involved. Five state reporting systems (CO, FL, MA, NY, and TN) ask for information about the function of the person(s) involved in or who contributed to the occurrence of the reported event. These systems differ considerably in terms of the information requested regarding who was involved. The categories of information required by each system regarding the role of the person involved in the event are shown in Table 5.4.

Table 5.4. Categories of Information Used to Specify the Role of the Person Involved in the Event

Role of Person Involved	CO	FL	MA	NY	TN
Physician				•	•
Nurse				•	•
Other staff			•	•	•
Pharmacist				•	•
Relation to client	•				
Who Assessed client	•				
Who was involved	•	•			

Two state systems (NY and TN) provide specific options regarding the functional role—physician, nurse, pharmacist or other staff member—of the person involved in the event. One system (CO) requests information about the relationship of the person involved in the event to the client. One system (CO) asks for a description of who assessed the client. Three systems (CO, FL, and MA) ask for a text description of the person(s) involved in the incident, including the person's role in the healthcare facility. Massachusetts also requests name, contact information, and role (aide, RN/LPN), and license number.

Dominant Cause Based on Preliminary Analysis. Six state reporting systems (CO, FL, GA-PHA, ME, MS and PA) ask for information about the dominant cause of the event. In Pennsylvania, reporters can provide as many "potential contributing factors" as applicable. Of the six state systems that ask for a description of the dominant cause, two (GA-PHA and PA) also require that a detailed root cause analysis be performed if indicated. Consequently, the dominant cause data element is the only information about the apparent cause of an event that is reported by four state systems. A reporting system was categorized as asking for information about dominant cause if this information was not requested as part of a root cause analysis.

The dominant cause of an adverse medical event is indicated by a menu choice and/or a narrative text. The Florida system asks for an identification of dominant cause in terms of an ICD-9 E code. The different options used by state reporting systems for specifying the dominant cause of an event are shown Table 5.5. All options except for the last ("Narrative") are picks from menus. The "Narrative" option indicates that the system requires a narrative description of the dominant cause of the event. Two state systems (ME and MS) require only a narrative description of the dominant cause of the event. Two other systems (CO and PA) require both a menu specification and a narrative description of the dominant cause of the event. The remaining systems require a selection from some subset of the options available for specifying the dominant cause of the event.

Table 5.5. Distribution of Categories of the Dominant Cause(s) of an Event Across State Systems

Dominant Cause	CO	FL	GA-PHA	ME	MS	PA
Communications			•			
Equipment			•			
Organization/management						•
Patient characteristics	•					•
Physical environment			•			
Policies/procedures	•		•			
Staff factors	•		•			•
Task factors	•					•
Team factors						•
Work environment						•
General	•	•				
Narrative	•			•	•	•

Risk Assessment. There are three components related to risk assessment: severity of the event, preventability of the event, and likelihood of recurrence of the event. Four state reporting systems (GA-PHA, MN, NJ and PA) ask for information about the severity of the adverse medical event. The event severity measures used by each of these systems are shown in Table 5.6. Two of these systems (GA-PHA and PA) use a version of the USP MedMARx Error Outcome Categories (U.S. Pharmacopeia, 2003). The MedMARx system provides a one-dimensional ranking of the severity of an event. Pennsylvania uses the full nine levels of severity used in MedMARx, where the least severe is "An event occurred but it did not reach the individual ("near miss" or "close call") because of active recovery efforts by caregivers" and the most severe is "An event occurred that contributed to or resulted in death." The Georgia PHA system uses five levels of severity, ranging from least severe ("An error occurred that may have contributed to or resulted in temporary harm to the patient and required initial or prolonged hospitalization") to most severe ("An error occurred that resulted in patient death"). Minnesota added a tenth level of severity to the MedMARx levels to reflect emotional injury.

Table 5.6. Event Severity Measures Used by Each of the State Systems

Severity Measure	GA-PHA	MN	NJ	PA
MedMARx	●	●		●
VHA			●	●

New Jersey uses 20 types of outcomes that roughly correspond to the three factors (extent of injury, length of stay, and level of care for remedy) that make up VHA severity categories. For example, level of care needed for remedy is measured through "additional laboratory testing or diagnostic imaging," "other additional diagnostic testing," "additional patient monitoring in current location," "visit to Emergency Department," "minor surgery," and "major surgery."

For some events (e.g., adverse drug events or ADEs), Pennsylvania uses the VHA prioritization scoring for close calls and adverse events, which is based on the actual or potential severity of the event (catastrophic, major, moderate, and minor) and the probability of recurrence (frequent, occasional, uncommon, and remote) (Department of Veterans Affairs, 2001). The resulting harm score indicates what type of response was required. For ADEs, resulting responses range from "to be determined" or "mild reaction requiring no treatment" to "death of the patient is directly related to ADR."

None of the systems investigated asked for information regarding the preventability of the event.

Narrative of the Event. Twenty state reporting systems explicitly require a textual narrative description of the event. Although it is not explicit in the information provided, we assume that Mississippi also requires some type of narrative or description of the event that includes, at a minimum, "causal factors, date and time of occurrence, and location of occurrence of the event." Neither Texas nor Kansas, both of which have aggregate reporting forms, requires narratives of the events, and neither does Nevada. Nevada is the only state that requires reporting of each reportable incident but does not require a narrative of what happened.

ANCILLARY INFORMATION

The IOM recommends that reports of adverse events include two pieces of ancillary information regarding each event: product information, in case some product or device was involved in the event, and patient information—in particular, the patient's age, gender, ethnicity, diagnosis, procedures, and comorbid conditions.

Product Information. Seven state reporting systems (CO, FL, MA, NJ, NY, PA, and TN) specifically ask for some type of product information.

The major categories of product information requested by the different state reporting systems are shown in Table 5.7. Five systems (CO, FL, MA, NJ, and PA) request some kind of information about the medical equipment involved in the event. Information requested about equipment includes the name of the manufacturer, model, and serial number. We also count information about medications as product information. Five systems (CO, NJ, NY, PA, and TN) request information about any medication that might have been involved in an event. This information can be used as the basis for describing medical events based on prescribing errors. The New York system requests information that would be particularly useful for this purpose since it collects information regarding the specific features of a prescription (i.e., medication name, dose, frequency, and route) that were intended and those that were actually written.

Table 5.7. Distribution of Categories of Product Information Across State Systems

Product Information	CO	FL	MA	NJ	NY	PA	TN
Equipment information	•	•	•	•		•	
Medication dosage					•	•	•
Intended dosage					•		
Medication frequency					•		•
Intended frequency					•		
Medication name	•			•	•	•	•
Intended medication name					•		
Medication route					•	•	•
Intended route					•		

Patient Information. Fourteen state reporting systems (CO, CT, FL, GA-PHA, GA-GDHR, ME, MA, MN, NV, NJ, NY, PA, TN, and UT) ask for some type of patient information. But, as shown in Table 5.8, the systems vary considerably in terms of what information about the patient is collected.

Table 5.8. Distribution of Categories of Patient Information Across State Systems

Patient information	CO	CT	FL	GA-PHA	GA-GDHR	ME	MA	MN	NV	NJ	NY	PA	TN	UT
Age/birthdate	•	•	•	•	•	•	•		•	•	•	•	•	•
Sex	•	•	•	•	•	•	•		•	•	•	•	•	•
Race/ethnicity										•			•	
Admit diagnosis		•	•	•	•	•				•	•		•	•
Discharge diagnosis														•
Procedures	•										•		•	

Patient information	CO	CT	FL	GA-PHA	GA-GDHR	ME	MA	MN	NV	NJ	NY	PA	TN	UT
Admission date	•	•	•		•		•			•	•	•		
Patient name		•	•		•		•							
Patient address		•	•						•	•				
Insurance			•											
Status before event	•				•		•	•		•		•		
Social security number		•												
Medical record/billing number		•			•					•			•	
Admission status											•			

The IOM recommends that information be collected about the patient's age, sex, ethnicity, diagnosis, procedures and comorbid conditions. All but one (MN) of the systems that require reporting of patient information ask for patient's age and sex. Only two systems (NJ and TN) currently collect information about the patient's race and ethnicity. Nine systems collect information about a patient's admission diagnosis, and one (UT) collects information about the patient's discharge diagnosis. Two of the systems that collect information about a patient's admission diagnosis (FL and NY) also ask for this information in terms of its ICD-9 code. Three state reporting systems (CO, NY, and TN) collect information about the procedures performed on the patient. New York asks that this procedure information be provided in terms of ICD-9 codes. None of the state reporting systems currently asks for information about a patient's comorbid conditions.

We found that a number of state reporting systems ask for patient information that is not specifically recommended in the IOM (2004) report. For example, four systems (CT, FL, GA-GDHR, and MA) ask for the patient's name. One system (FL) also asks for the patient's address and insurance status. Six systems (CO, GA-GDHR, MA, MN, NJ, and PA) ask for the patient's status before the event. One system (CT) asks for the patient's social security number, and four systems (CT, GA-GDHR, NJ, and

TN) ask for the patient's medical record or billing number. Finally, one system (NJ) asks for the patent's status upon admission.

DETAILED CAUSAL ANALYSIS

The IOM recommends that a formal RCA be performed if it is warranted by the severity of the event. If an RCA is performed, the IOM recommends that the following information be reported regarding the results of the analysis:

- technical, organizational, and human factors

- recovery from near misses

- corrective actions taken

- patient outcome/functional status

- similar case recently investigated.

Root Causes. There are two major systems for reporting findings of root causes analysis used by states. One is the Eindhoven Classification Model (Battles et al., 1998). This system looks at the potential causes from three perspectives, which represent three different causal domains:

- technical factors (equipment, software and forms)

- organizational factors (policies, procedures and protocols)

- human factors (knowledge-based, rule-based and skill based human performance factors).

The second is VHA's National Center for Patient Safety (NCPS) scheme (Bagian et al., 2001). VHA NCPS focuses on six causal areas:

- human factors--communication

- human factors--training

- human factors--fatigue/scheduling

- environment/equipment

- rules/policies/procedures

- barriers (safeguards).

Table 5.9 summarizes the states' use of root cause coding schemes. The Georgia PHA system requires reporters to specify whether the root cause was a technical, organizational, or a human factor (drawing on the Eindhoven scheme).

Four reporting systems (MN, NJ, NY, and TN) ask the reporter to specify one or more contributing factors that fall within one or more of the six causal areas delineated in the NPFS scheme. Nevada asks reporters to select up to four different contributing factors that fall under any of three Eindhoven (Human factors, Organization/management, and Technical) domains or two NCPS (Environment/equipment and Information/communication) domains. Pennsylvania asks reporters to indicate up to three root causes from among 19 JCAHO categories, which are similar to, but not exactly the same as, the NCPS categories and the 20 Eindhoven (Medical Version) categories. Utah and Wyoming roughly follow the NCPS format in that an RCA is to be completed by the facility, with a narrative of the findings to be submitted to the state.

Table 5.9. Root Cause Coding Schemes Used in Nine State Systems

	GA-PHA	MN	NV	NJ	NY	PA	TN	UT	WY
Eindhoven	•								
VNA NCPS		•		•	•		•		
VHA NCPS + Eindhoven			•						
Eindhoven (Medical) + JCAHO						•			
Narrative								•	•

Causal Analysis: Recovery from Near Misses. None of the state reporting systems studied asked for information regarding the recovery factors that can occur at each point when there are near misses.

Causal Analysis: Corrective Actions Taken. Eighteen state reporting systems (CO, CT, FL, GA-PHA, GA-GDHR, KS, ME, MA, MN, NV, NJ, NY, PA, RI, TN, TX, UT, and WY) ask for information about the type of corrective actions taken after the reported event. Since only nine reporting systems (those shown in Table 5.9) require that an RCA be performed, the information about corrective actions in the other nine systems (CO, CT, FL, FL, GA-GDHR, KS, ME, MA, RI, and TX) is not actually part of an RCA.

Table 5.10. Distribution of Requirements for Information Regarding Corrective Actions Taken After an Event

Corrective Actions Taken	CO	CT	FL	GA-PHA	GA-GDHR	KS	ME	MA	MN	NV	NJ	NY	PA	RI	TN	TX	UT	WY
Action plan		•											•				•	•
Action taken (general)	•		•	•	•	•	•	•	•	•	•	•	•	•	•			
Action taken (specific)	•					•				•		•	•		•			
Evaluation		•					•		•			•			•	•		
Plan/policy in place												•			•			
Recommendations				•														
No action necessary													•					

The categories of information about corrective actions that are required by each state system are shown in Table 5.10. Four systems ask for corrective actions in terms of an action plan. Most systems (all but CT, TX, UT, and WY) ask for a general, narrative description of the corrective actions that were taken. Six systems (CO, KS, NV, NY, PA, and TN) ask for information about corrective actions in terms of specific options, which include "Equipment modification," "Environmental change," "Staff education," and "Policy/procedure change." Other corrective action options include an evaluation of the status of the situation before and after corrective action were taken (CT, ME, MN, NY, TN, and TX) and a description of the corrective policy or plan that that was put into place after the event (NY and TN). The Georgia PHA system asks for specific recommendations regarding corrective actions that should be taken in response to the event. These options include making a change in communications, equipment, environment, or policies and procedures. Finally, Pennsylvania allows an indication that no corrective action was deemed necessary.

Causal Analysis: Patient Outcome/Functional Status. Seven state systems (CO, MA, NJ, NY, PA, RI, and TN) request information regarding the status of the patient after an event. The classes of information about patient outcomes that are required by each state system are shown in Table 5.11.

Table 5.11. Distribution of Requirements for Reporting Information Regarding the Outcome of an Event

Outcome	CO	MA	NJ	NY	PA	RI	TN
Additional care/treatment	•		•		•		
Additional cost					•		
Additional monitoring	•						
Patient state	•	•	•		•	•	
Non-patient outcome		•	•	•	•		•

Three systems (CO, NJ, and PA) ask whether additional care or treatment was necessitated by the event. One system (PA) asks whether there was additional cost incurred by the event. One system (CO) asks whether additional monitoring was required. Five systems (CO, MA, NJ, PA, and RI) ask specifically for information about the patient's state following an event. Rhode Island asks for this information in narrative form. The remaining systems ask for this information in terms of menu options, such as "Loss of limb(s)," "Loss of digit(s)," "Loss of body part(s)," and "Loss of bodily function(s)," "Visit to the emergency hospital," and "Death." Finally, five systems (MA, NJ, NY, PA, and TN) ask for information about outcomes that are not directly related to the state of the patient, such as property damage.

Causal Analysis: Similar Case Recently Investigated. Only one state system (CO) requests information about similar events that were recently investigated. The Colorado system requiring reporting of this information in the form of estimates of the number of occurrences of events similar to the one that occurred. If the event was a "Life-Threatening Transfusion Error/Reaction," the person filing the report would be asked "How many Life-Threatening Transfusion Error/Reaction Occurrences have been reported by your facility in the last 6 months"?

LESSONS LEARNED

Four state reporting systems (KS, NV, NY, and PA) ask for information about any safety lessons that were learned from the event. These systems solicit this information in the form of a narrative description of "lessons learned" or "recommendations for system improvement" made as a result of the event.

OTHER ELEMENTS

All data elements on state reporting forms that could not be categorized in terms of the IOM-recommended elements were grouped together as "Other Data Elements." Approximately 400 data elements from the report forms of 18 different reporting systems could not be categorized in terms of the IOM categories shown in Table 2.1. The kind of information captured as "Other Data Elements" ranges from information about the healthcare facility reporting the event to whether or not an autopsy was performed in case of a death. Some of the categories of the information requested as "Other Data Elements" are shown in Table 5.12, which also shows how these categories of information are distributed across the state reporting systems.

Table 5.12. Distribution of Requirements for Reporting "Other" Information That Is Not Recommended by the IOM

Categories of other information	CO	CT	FL	GA-PHA	GA-GDHR	KS	ME	MA	MN	MS	NV	NJ	NY	PA	TN	TX	UT	WA
Additional information	•	•				•					•		•	•	•	•	•	
Autopsy performed		•	•															
Facility information	•	•	•		•	•	•	•	•		•	•	•		•	•	•	•
Others notified	•	•	•					•		•								
Name/title of person reporting	•	•	•		•	•	•	•			•		•					•
Report submission date	•	•				•	•	•			•		•				•	
Discovery date/time	•	•		•	•		•		•		•	•	•				•	
Status before event	•																	

Table 5.12 shows only a subset of all the non-recommended information provided by the different state systems. Nine systems (CO, CT, KS, NV, NY, PA, TN, TX, and UT) request "Additional information" about an event that is not recommended by the IOM. This "Additional information" category includes the names of participants in the RCA, whether safety precautions were in place, whether the event qualifies as a JCAHO sentinel event, and whether charges were filed against an assailant. Two systems (CT and FL) ask whether an autopsy was performed in the case of a death.

A very common type of information provided in reports, but not recommended by the IOM, is information about the facility at which the adverse medical event occurred. Fifteen systems (CO, CT, FL, GA-GDHR, KS, ME, MA, MN, NV, NJ, NY, TN, TX, UT, and WA, and) request "Facility information," such as the name, address, and type of facility (e.g., hospital, ambulatory surgical center).

Five systems (CO, CT, FL, MA, and MI) request information regarding "Others notified" about the event. Options provided regarding "Others notified" include family, police, medical examiner, physician, and ombudsman.

Several systems require information that is quite similar but not equivalent to the information recommended by IOM. For example, ten systems (CO, CT, FL, GA-GDHR, KS, ME, MA, NJ, TN, and WA) request information about the name and/or title of the person reporting the event. IOM recommends reporting only the function of those who were actually involved in the event. Eight systems (CO, CT, KS, ME, MA, NJ, TN, and UT) ask when the report was submitted, and ten systems (CO, CT, GA-PHA, GA-GDHR, ME, MN, NJ, NY, TN, and UT) request information about when the event was discovered. IOM recommends reporting only when the event occurred. Finally, one system (CO) asks for information about the status of a patient before the event occurred.

SUMMARY

Existing state adverse medical event reporting systems vary significantly in terms of what information is reported about adverse medical events and how that information is reported—that is, in the values of the data elements recorded. The existing variability in the information reported indicates that collecting national data regarding the incidence and circumstances surrounding the occurrence of adverse medical events will be difficult, if not impossible, without extensive efforts to develop a reporting system that all states can and will use.

6. EXISTING MEDICAL STANDARDS APPLICABLE TO ADVERSE EVENT REPORTING

Adverse event reports contain information that can be used by safety experts to detect trends in the types of adverse medical events that occur and the causes of these events. But to use data regarding adverse medical events most effectively, the information in the reports from the different states and accreditation agencies must be available to safety experts in a standard form. Without a standard for the form of the data to be reported by the different sources, it will be difficult to assemble those data into a central repository for analysis.

As noted in the previous chapter, we found very little use of standard coding methods in state adverse medical event reports. The only standard coding scheme currently in use seems to be the ICD-9 diagnostic codes. Florida uses ICD-9 E codes to describe the dominant cause of an event. Florida and New York use ICD-9 to describe a patient's admitting diagnosis, and New York uses ICD-9 to describe procedure information. Moreover, our survey showed that states were not recoding any information based on text reports.

Thus, we set out to evaluate existing standards for reporting health information in other contexts—that is, outside the context of patient safety and the reporting of adverse medical events. Our aim was to assess the extent to which the information in adverse medical event reports could be coded using the standards for reporting health information that are used in other contexts. More specifically, we attempted to determine whether existing health information standards could be applied to each of the IOM-recommended data elements for adverse medical event reporting. This chapter describes our approach and the results of that assessment.

IDENTIFICATION OF EXISTING STANDARDS FOR REPORTING HEALTH INFORMATION

In consultation with our AHRQ project officer, we decided to review the 27 standards identified by the Consolidated Health Informatics (CHI) initiative. CHI, conducted under the leadership of the U.S. Office of Management and Budget, is an effort to identify a portfolio of already existing interoperability standards for health information (health vocabulary and messaging) that would allow all federal agencies involved in the "health enterprise" to speak the same language based on common enterprise-wide business and information technology architectures.[16]

In the remainder of this chapter, we review the standards identified (and in many cases approved) by CHI. The standards are organized around the target domains (representing administrative or clinical procedures related to the delivery of healthcare). From this review, we identified 23 health informatics standards that could potentially be used for one or more IOM-recommended domains. These 23 health informatics standards, along with the respective domains our analysis indicates they may apply to, are represented in Table 6.1. As discussed below, we also reviewed an additional four CHI-identified standards but did not find them to be applicable to any of the IOM-recommended data elements.

---

[16] www.whitehouse.gov/omb/egov/c-3-6-chi.html (last accessed December 25, 2005).

Table 6.1. Relationship of Health Information Standards to IOM Elements

IOM-Recommended Elements	HL7 2.3+ Messaging	LOINC Lab Result Names	HL7 2.4+ Demographics	HL7 2.x Units	HL7 2.3.1+ Immunizations	HL7 2.4+ Clinical Encounters	HL7 CDA 1.0-2000 Text Based Reports	SNOMED CT Lab Result Contents	SNOMED CT Non-Lab Intervention	SNOMED CT Anatomy	SNOMED CT Diagnosis	SNOMED CT Nursing	LOINC Laboratory Test Order Names	HIPAA Transactions and Code Set	HL7 2.4 Special Populations	NDF-RT Drug Classification	LOINC Product Labels	FDA/NDC Drug Product	FDA/CDER Package	FDA Established Name and FDA UNII	RxNorm SCD	FDA/CDER Dosage Form	EPA Substance Registry
Role of person who discovered event	●		●	●	●	●	●					●			●								
How event was discovered	●		●	●	●	●	●					●			●								
Event type (what happened)	●		●	●	●	●	●			●	●				●								
Where in the care process the event was discovered	●		●	●	●	●	●		●						●								
When the event occurred	●		●	●	●	●	●		●			●			●								
Function of those involved	●		●	●	●	●	●		●						●								
Dominant cause	●		●	●	●	●	●								●								
Risk assessment																							
Severity of event	●		●	●	●	●	●				●	●			●								
Preventability of event	●		●	●	●	●	●					●			●								
Likelihood of recurrence	●		●	●	●	●	●					●			●								
Narrative of the event	●				●	●	●																
Ancillary Information																							
Product information	●		●	●	●	●	●	●	●	●	●	●	●	●	●	●	●	●	●	●	●	●	●
Patient information	●	●	●	●	●	●	●		●			●		●	●								
Causal Analysis																							
Technical, organizational, and human factors	●		●	●	●	●	●					●			●								●
Recovery from for near misses	●		●		●	●	●					●			●								
Corrective actions taken	●		●		●	●	●					●			●								
Patient outcome/status	●	●	●		●	●	●				●	●			●								
If similar case recently	●		●		●	●	●					●			●								
Lessons learned from the event	●		●		●	●	●					●			●								

CHI-Approved Standards

In this section, we discuss the relevance of the CHI standards to the adverse medical event report information represented by the data elements shown in Table 6.1.

General Messaging Standards. Messaging standards include standards for order entry, scheduling, medical record/image management, patient administration, observation reporting, financial management, patient care, and public health notification. The National Committee on Vital and Health Statistics (NCVHS) recommended adopting HL7 version 2.3+ as the approach to developing messaging standards for healthcare data with expectations to move quickly to version 3. HL7 is a Standards Developing Organization that is accredited by the American National Standards Institute. It is made up of providers, vendors, payers, consultants, government groups, and others.[17] The first column in Table 6.1 reflects our judgment that the general messaging standards of HL7 2.3+ could, with appropriate modifications and extensions, be applied to all the IOM-recommended data elements.

Messaging Standards: Retail Pharmacy Transactions. This standard covers the electronic transfer of prescription data between retail pharmacies and those who write new prescriptions, changes, refills, status notifications, and cancellation notifications. NCVHS recommended the adoption of the National Council for Prescription Drug Programs SCRIPT data transmission standard.[18] Since the NCVS standard applies to transactions between prescribers and retail pharmacies, we do not believe that the standard is applicable to reports of adverse medical events that occur in hospitals.

Messaging Standards: Connectivity. The Institute of Electrical and Electronics Engineers 1073 series standard provides an internal messaging standard for communication among medical devices. It has

---

[17] www.whitehouse.gov/omb/egov/documents/domain2.doc (last accessed December 15, 2005.)

[18] www.whitehouse.gov/omb/egov/documents/domain3.doc (last accessed December 15, 2005.)

received a conditional recommendation from HHS, with the caveat that it only applies within an agency. This standard is deployed in Europe, but is only in investigational deployment in the United States.[19]

Currently, we find this standard to have no obvious relevance to coding any IOM-recommended adverse medical event information.

Messaging Standards: Image Information and Workstations. The DICOM standard is a messaging standard for images that allows images and associated diagnostic information to be retrieved and transferred from various manufacturers' devices, as well as from medical staff workstations.[20] DICOM has two parts: information objects (how images and image-related information are encoded) and services (how information objects are exchanged between instruments).[21] Because these standards concern machine-to-machine messaging, DICOM has no apparent relevance to coding the IOM data elements.

Laboratory Results Names. The Logical Observation Identifiers Names and Codes (LOINC) system provides complete and flexible terminology for naming laboratory results.[22] It has been widely accepted in both the public and private sectors. The Regenstrief Institute, Inc., owns LOIN4C.[23] Because LOINC provides standard codes for drug-related laboratory results, LOINC for lab results is likely to be relevant to coding product information associated with adverse events.

Demographics. HL7 version 2.4+ was adopted as the standard storing specific patient demographic data, to be used for various purposes but primarily for unique patient identification.[24] While the focus of HL7 2.4+ is patient demographic data, which would apply mainly to patient

---

[19]www.whitehouse.gov/omb/egov/documents/domain4.doc (last accessed December 15, 2005).

[20]www.medical.nema.org (last accessed December 15, 2005).

[21]www.whitehouse.gov/omb/egov/documents/domain5.doc (last accessed December 15, 2005).

[22]www.whitehouse.gov/omb/egov/documents/domain1.doc (last accessed December 15, 2005).

[23]www.regenstrief.org/loinc (last accessed December 15, 2005).

[24]www.whitehouse.gov/omb/egov/documents/demo_full_public.doc (last accessed December 15, 2005).

information, the standard includes coding schemes that could apply to all IOM-recommended data elements.

Units. The Units standard is a sub-domain of another standard, Laboratory Result Content. This standard is used to define common units of measure, such as Celsius or mg/ml, which are to be combined with a numeric value to express a result. HL7 version 2.X was adopted as the standard for this information.[25] The focus of HL7 2.X is patient demographic data, which would apply mainly to patient information. But, like HL7 2.4+, HL7 2.X includes coding schemes that apply to all IOM-recommended data elements.

Immunizations. HL7's immunization registry terminology—specifically the CVX (clinical vaccine formulation) and MVX (manufacturer) codes—have been adopted as the data standard for the storage and exchange of immunization information.[26] These immunization standards, listed as HL7 2.3.1+ in Table 6.1, apply to product information and patient information. But, again, the standard includes coding schemes that, with modifications, could be applied to all IOM-recommended data elements.

Clinical Encounters. An encounter between a patient and a healthcare provider serves as a focal point linking clinical, administrative, and financial information. HL7 Version 2.4+ is the standard for clinical encounters.[27] Because these encounters may occur in many different settings within a healthcare facility, HL7 2.4+ would be particularly well suited to coding information concerning where in the care process an adverse medical event occurred. We believe the standard could also be applied to coding when the event occurred and the function of those involved in the event. As with all other

---

[25]www.whitehouse.gov/omb/egov/documents/lrc_and_units_full_public.doc (last accessed December 15, 2005).

[26]www.whitehouse.gov/omb/egov/documents/immun_full_public.doc (last accessed December 15, 2005).

[27]www.whitehouse.gov/omb/egov/documents/encounter_full_public.doc (last accessed December 15, 2005).

implementations of HL7, the standard includes coding schemes that could be applied to all TOM-recommended data elements.

Text-Based Reports. The scope of this standard is to identify standards and terminologies that can be used to define the architecture and syntax for clinical document messages. HL7's CDA (Clinical Document Architecture) Release 1.0-2000 has been identified as the standard that defines the messaging architecture and syntax of clinical text documents.[28] This standard is likely to be most applicable to the coding of the narrative description of adverse events. This standard could be also used to code lessons learned, which is typically entered as text, as well as any other information about an event that is entered as text.

Laboratory Result Content. The primary focus of this standard concerns the exchange of laboratory test results among healthcare facilities. Laboratory results have four basic parts: the result itself, the result units (see Units above) if applicable, normal range or indicator flags, and any comments associated with the results. The Systematized Nomenclature of Medicine Clinical Terms (SNOMED CT) has been adopted as the standard for the exchange of laboratory test results. SNOMED has made the content and terminology of its standards available through the Unified Medical Language System (UMLS) at the National Library of Medicine.[29] The development of SNOMED CT for laboratory result content is likely to make it applicable to coding patient information.

Non-Laboratory Interventions and Procedures. This standard describes specific non-laboratory interventions and procedures performed and/or delivered. Interventions represent purposeful activities performed in the provision of healthcare. Procedures are defined as concepts that represent the purposeful activities performed in the provision of healthcare. SNOMED CT has been identified and adopted by

---

[28] www.whitehouse.gov/omb/egov/documents/text_full_public.doc (last accessed December 15, 2005).

[29]www.whitehouse.gov/omb/egov/documents/lrc_and_units_full_public.doc (last accessed December 15, 2005).

HHS for this standard. It is a dynamic and continually evolving standard; there is, however, some concern about the speed in which new and emerging technologies are incorporated.[30]

The development of SNOMED CT for non-laboratory interventions and procedures will make it applicable mainly to coding patient information. We believe this standard can also be used to code information relevant to where in the care process an event occurred, when the event occurred, the function of those involved in the event, and product information related to the event.

Anatomy/Physiology. A combination of SNOMED CT and the National Cancer Institute Thesaurus (not shown in Table 1) has been identified as the standard for describing anatomy. No standard has been recommended for physiology. This resource covers vocabulary for clinical care, translational and basic research, and public information and administrative activities.[31] The anatomical coding scheme in SNOMED makes it applicable to coding aspects of the type of event that occurred, such as the site of a wrong-site surgery. We believe this standard could also be used to code patient information.

Diagnosis and Problem List. SNOMED CT has been adopted as the standard for describing all medical, nursing, dental, social, preventive, and psychiatric events and issues that are relevant to a given patient's healthcare. These include signs, symptoms, and defined conditions.[32] As with SNOMED CT for laboratory results, we believe that SNOMED CT for diagnosis and other problems will be applicable to coding patient information, type of event, risk assessment: severity of event, and root cause: outcome of an event.

Nursing. SNOMED CT is has been adopted as the standard terminology used to identify, classify, and name the delivery of nursing care.

---

[30]www.whitehouse.gov/omb/egov/documents/iandp_nonlab_full_public.do c (last accessed December 15, 2005).

[31]www.whitehouse.gov/omb/egov/documents/aandp_full_public.doc (last accessed December 15, 2005).

[32]www.whitehouse.gov/omb/egov/documents/dxandprob_full_public.doc (last accessed December 15, 2005).

Within this large set of activities, sub-domains have been identified; these sub-domains are derived from the Nursing Process and American Nursing Association-recognized Nursing Minimum Data Set, with an emphasis on nursing assessment, diagnosis, interventions, and outcomes of nursing care.[33]

The SNOMED coding scheme for nursing care is applicable to coding many of the IOM-recommended data elements because this standard covers so many aspects of the care process. We believe that the SNOMED CT Nursing standard could be used to code the role of person who discovered event (such as a nurse), how the event was discovered (as when a family member brings the event to nurse's attention), when the event occurred, patient information, type of event, risk assessment: severity of event, risk assessment: preventability of event, risk assessment: likelihood of recurrence, product information, causal analysis: technical, organizations, and human factors, causal analysis: recovery from near misses, causal analysis: corrective actions taken, and causal analysis: patient outcome/functional status.

Laboratory Test Order Names. LOINC has been adopted as the approved standard representation of the names of laboratory tests associated with an order within a computer system.[34] Table 6.1 shows that LOINC for test orders, like LOINC for test results, is likely to be most relevant to coding patient information associated with adverse events.

Billing/Financial. Billing and financial standards are used to implement the electronic exchange of health-related information needed to perform billing and administrative functions in the healthcare enterprise. The standards specified in the regulations associated with the Health Insurance Portability and Accounting Act (HIPAA) are the approved transactions and codes set. These include ICD-9; the National Drug Codes (NDC) medication codes, maintained by the Food and Drug

---

[33] www.whitehouse.gov/omb/egov/documents/nursing_full_public.doc (last accessed December 15, 2005).

[34] www.whitehouse.gov/omb/egov/documents/ltornm_full_public.doc (last accessed December 15, 2005).

Administration (FDA); the Healthcare Common Procedure Coding System (HCPCS) codes, maintained by the Centers for Medicare and Medicaid Services (CMS); the Current Procedural Terminology (CPT-4) diagnostic codes, maintained by the American Medical Association; the Current Dental Terminology (CDT) codes, maintained by the American Dental Association; the ABC Coding Solutions and the Diagnosis Related Groups (DRG) codes, also maintained by CMS.[35] The HIPAA standard could be used to code patient information (particularly diagnosis and procedure information) and product information.

Medications: Special Populations. HL7 version 2.4 gender, race, and ethnicity codes have been recommended and adopted for identifying subgroups of the population using medications for the treatment or prevention of medical conditions. The standard can be used to code the difference in the safety and effectiveness of these products. They are also consistent with the demographics standard.[36] The HL7 2.4 standard codes patient demographic data, which would apply mainly to patient information in adverse event reporting. But the standard includes coding schemes that apply to all IOM-recommended data elements.

Medications: Drug Classifications. The National Drug File Reference Terminology (NDF-RT) classification scheme, developed by the Veterans Administration for the areas of physiological effect and mechanism of action, provides a hierarchical coding scheme for categorizing each medication. Coding categories include mechanism of action, physiologic effects, intended therapeutic use, chemical structures, pharmacological properties, and FDA-approved indications.[37] The CHI Medications group recommended that the full Council encourage the FDA to improve and revise NDC codes and NDC code generation

[35]www.whitehouse.gov/omb/egov/documents/billing_full_public.doc (last accessed December 15, 2005).
[36]www.whitehouse.gov/omb/egov/documents/med_asummary_full_public.doc (last accessed December 15, 2005).
[37]www.whitehouse.gov/omb/egov/documents/med_asummary_full_public.doc (last accessed December 15, 2005).

processes to address problem areas. NDF-RT can be used to code product information.

Medications: Structured Product Label. LOINC is the approved standard for the submission, review, storage, dissemination, and access to product labeling information. The purpose of the LOINC standards for product labels is to provide labeling information electronically, in a human readable text format that can be exchanged across systems.[38] The LOINC product labels standard can be used to code product information, particularly information about medication products involved in an adverse event.

Medications: Drug Product. The FDA NDC standard enables the healthcare sector to share information regarding drug products. The NDC serves as a universal product identifier for medications used by humans.[39] The FDA NDC standard can be used to code product information regarding medications involved in an adverse event.

Medications: Package. The FDA's Center for Drug Evaluation and Research (CDER) Data Standards Manual consists of standardized nomenclature monographs that have been reviewed and approved by the CDER Nomenclature Standards Committee. The purpose of this standard is to enable the healthcare sector to share information regarding drug packages. The Data Standards Manual was identified as the approved standard.[40] The FDA CDER Package standard, like the FDA NDC, can be used to a limited extent to code product information regarding medications involved in an adverse event.

Medications: Active Ingredients. The FDA's Established Name for active ingredient and its Unique Ingredient Identifier (UNII) codes are the standards that enable the healthcare sector to share information regarding the active ingredients in medication. An active ingredient is

---

[38] www.whitehouse.gov/omb/egov/documents/medSPL_full_public.doc (last accessed December 25, 2005).

[39] www.whitehouse.gov/omb/egov/documents/medprod_full_public.doc (last accessed December 15, 2005).

[40]www.whitehouse.gov/omb/egov/documents/medpkg_full_public.doc (last accessed December 15, 2005).

defined as the substance responsible for the effects of a medication. Established Names may consist of up to 3 fields: Active ingredient, dosage form, and route of administration. UNII codes are unique ingredient identifiers based on molecular structure, manufacturing process, and/or other characteristics.[41] The FDA Established Name and FDA UNII can be used to code product information regarding medications involved in an adverse event, particularly as these relate to dosage form and route of administration.

Medications: Clinical Drugs. The Semantic Clinical Drug (SCD) of RxNorm has been adopted as the approved standard for identifying the active ingredients in medications. The purpose of the standards was to allow the mapping of proprietary systems to a standard clinical drug nomenclature.[42] The RxNorm SCD standard can be used to code product information regarding medications, particularly as these relate to the distinction between generic and proprietary drugs.

Medications: Manufactured Dosage Form. The FDA CDER Dosage Form standard enables the sharing of information regarding drug dosage forms. A manufactured dosage form is the way of identifying a drug in its physical form. In determining these forms, one includes such factors as physical appearance of the drug product, physical form of the drug product prior to dispensing it to the patient, the way the product is administered, frequency of dosing, and how pharmacists and other health professionals might recognize and handle the product.[43] The FDA CDER Dosage Form standard can be used to code product information regarding medications involved in an adverse event.

Genes and Proteins. The Human Gene Nomenclature (HUGN) sponsored by the Human Genome Organization allows the healthcare sector to exchange information regarding the role of genes in biomedical research

---

[41]www.whitehouse.gov/omb/egov/documents/med_ingred_full_public.doc (last accessed December 15, 2005).

[42]www.whitehouse.gov/omb/egov/documents/med_clindrug_full_public.doc (last accessed December 15, 2005).

[43]www.whitehouse.gov/omb/egov/documents/med_dose_full_public.doc (last accessed December 15, 2005).

and healthcare, using a single unambiguous genetic nomenclature.[44] We can find no obvious application of HUGN to coding any of the IOM-recommended information regarding an adverse medical event.

Chemicals. The Environmental Protection Agency's Substance Registry System (EPA SRS) has been conditionally adopted as the standard for coding chemicals of importance to healthcare outside of medications, such as those found in the workplace or the environment.[45] The EPA SRS would be most relevant to coding product information. However, we believe this standard could also be used to code information about the root cause of an adverse medical event (causal analysis: technical, organizations, and human factors), particularly when the root cause involves a chemical substance in the environment.

STANDARDS NEEDED WHERE NO STANDARD HAS YET BEEN IDENTIFIED

Disability. A standard for coding disability would be used to describe disability terms that are used in the healthcare sector. It could potentially be used by agencies such as CMS for payment, surveys, public quality reports, external quality monitoring, internal quality monitoring, eligibility determinations, and policy development. No standard is being recommended for adoption at this time.[46]

History and Physical. This standard would define terminology to identify, classify, and name the components incorporated into a patient's medical history and the physical exam process performed by a practitioner. No recommendations for this standard have been made. The work has been deferred.[47]

Medical Devices and Supplies. This standard would be used to inventory medical devices and supplies and to document their use by

---

[44]http://www.whitehouse.gov/omb/egov/documents/genes_public_full.doc (last accessed December 15, 2005).

[45]www.whitehouse.gov/omb/egov/documents/chem_full_public.doc (last accessed December 15, 2005).

[46]www.whitehouse.gov/omb/egov/documents/disability_full_public.doc (last accessed December 15, 2005).

[47]www.whitehouse.gov/omb/egov/documents/handp_full_public.doc (lat accessed December 14, 2005).

health services establishments, as well as to regulate medical device and supply availability and utilization in the community by public health agencies. There is a recommendation to encourage two different device-naming standards—the Global Medical Device Nomenclature and the Universal Medical Device Nomenclature System—to merge. The resulting terminology could then be reevaluated and/or adopted.[48]

Multimedia. This standard would be used to combine data from multiple media (e.g., images, photos, audios, videos, faxes, etc.) into patient records with the objective of ensuring interoperability and information exchange among agencies. No recommendation for such a standard has currently been made.[49]

Population Health. The scope of this standard involves enumerating code sets used to report data to public health entities and for the purpose of assembling population health statistics that were not specifically identified under other standards identified above. No standard has been recommended. Work is continuing. It has been noted that in some circumstances, population health data are identical to clinical data, such as reporting infectious disease cases to public health departments or reporting cancer rapid case ascertainment and other disease registry information to appropriate state registries.[50]

SUMMARY

This chapter describes federal standards for the exchange of electronic information regarding health and healthcare. Such federal standards are needed to provide a foundation for both research and effective administration in the vast bureaucracies that govern the delivery of healthcare and assess quality, efficacy, cost, and other

---

[48]www.whitehouse.gov/omb/egov/documents/supplies_full_public.doc (last accessed December 15, 2005).

[49]www.whitehouse.gov/omb/egov/documents/multimedia_I_full_public.doc (last accessed December 15, 2005).

[50]www.whitehouse.gov/omb/egov/documents/population_full_public.doc (last accessed December 15, 2005).

outcomes of healthcare. We have argued in previous chapters that similar standards would be useful in identifying patterns in the occurrence and characteristics of adverse medical events, and the results of the CHI initiative indicate that developing relevant standards is feasible. Indeed, our analysis suggests that efforts to develop standards for reporting adverse medical events can build on the CHI standards.

Existing standards can be used to code much of the IOM-recommended information regarding adverse medical events. Many of the detailed standards already exist for particular data elements, such as patient and product information. Standards for other elements can be developed in the context of existing standards (such as SNOMED and LOINC) through the efforts of organizing groups, such as HL7. We conclude that it will not be necessary to develop a special set of standards for the coding of information about adverse medical events. Standards for coding the information in adverse event reports already exist or are being developed within the existing framework of other standardization efforts (HL7). The process of standardizing the information in adverse medical event reports would be largely a matter of deciding which of the existing standards to use for this purpose.

7. DESIGN AND IMPLEMENTATION OF AN ADVERSE MEDICAL EVENTS REPORTING SYSTEM: THE VIEWS OF PATIENT SAFETY EXPERTS

To understand current patterns of adverse medical events and reduce their frequency, researchers, healthcare administrators, and policymakers need data that permit comparisons over time and across healthcare institutions—both within and across the 50 states. To collect ideas about how systems that permit such comparisons might be structured and implemented, RAND assembled a panel of the nation's foremost experts on patient safety assurance systems to begin to identify and define the essential features of an ideal adverse medical event reporting system and to consider how such a system might be administered to ensure that data regarding adverse medical events are collected using objective, systematic procedures and that the entity receiving and/or housing the data is independent of influence from healthcare providers and payers. In this chapter, we summarize the views of the panelists and discuss their implications for the design and management of adverse event reporting systems.

DETERMINING WHICH ADVERSE MEDICAL EVENTS SHOULD BE REPORTED

In an April 2005 Web conference organized by RAND, the panelists began with a discussion of the concept of medical error, with a view toward determining which errors should be reported to an adverse medical event reporting system. In particular, the panel discussed whether an adverse medical event reporting system should be designed to collect and store information about every conceivable error that occurs within a healthcare facility or only those errors that actually harm patients.

The panelists noted that the simple category of medical error is so broad that it encompasses events that harm patients, events that almost harm patients (i.e., near misses), and events that do not come close to harming patients but nevertheless should not occur within healthcare facilities. Also, several panelists noted that the number of errors that do not actually harm patients could potentially be so large, and the reporting of them so subjective, that it would be virtually impossible to capture details about them consistently across the states, even if every state were using the identical adverse medical event reporting system. Consequently, the panel agreed that the adverse medical event reports should focus only on events that cause harm to patients. The consensus was that the 27 "never events" endorsed by NQF in 2002, or something closely resembling them, was a reasonable place to start in identifying the adverse medical events that should form the core of an ideal event reporting system.

In reaching this conclusion, several panelists noted that healthcare facilities face a wide range of internal and external audiences that look to the various institutional reporting systems maintained by such facilities to provide them with quite different kinds of information. For instance, internal groups in healthcare facilities, such as administrators and members of the medical staff, need information that may differ considerably from that needed by external groups, such as accreditation and regulatory organizations (e.g., JCAHO, the FDA, and state departments of health). The latter groups are concerned not only about preventing adverse medical events but also about the much broader issue of the overall quality of healthcare. Moreover, the concerns of such entities extend well beyond the boundaries of individual healthcare organizations—even though such institutions may themselves be large and complex enough to be interested in cross-site comparisons of the occurrence of adverse medical events.

As a result, the panelists thought it critical that the state-based reporting systems used to capture data regarding adverse medical events be very clearly circumscribed and limited in scope so as to maximize the chances that such systems would be adopted and implemented in all states. Indeed, the panel cited the challenge of standardizing anything across healthcare institutions within a single state, much less across healthcare facilities in all states, as yet another reason for limiting the information reported to adverse medical event reporting systems to only those events that cause harm to patients. The panel's recommendations to use the NQF never events as a basis for the development of adverse event reporting systems and to focus on events that cause harm to patients are, to a considerable extent, consistent with current practices.

IDENTIFYING IMPORTANT ELEMENTS OF ADVERSE EVENTS

The next issue addressed by the panel was what categories of information—that is, what data elements regarding adverse medical events—should be recorded and reported to a state-based adverse medical event reporting system. Important elements might include not only a description of the adverse medical event but also such factors as the role of the healthcare personnel (e.g., physician, nurse) involved in the event, patient characteristics (e.g., age, gender), and other data that would provide a full description of the event; the factors that contributed to the event; and the consequences of the event.

Panelists readily agreed that simply reporting the outcome of adverse medical events was inadequate because such an approach would frustrate any efforts to use the information in these state-based reporting systems to learn what *not* to do while treating patients in healthcare facilities. Instead, all agreed that the information reported about the adverse medical event should start with "the end"— the event that harmed a patient—and work backward to capture as much information as possible about the complete chain of events that led up to the harmful outcome. Such a process would entail an RCA.

None of the panelists was prepared during the Web conference, however, to list "on the fly" the specific data elements that would make up the core of an ideal patient safety tracking system. Panelists readily agreed though, that, to the extent possible, reports regarding adverse medical events should use terminology that has already been standardized, such as that for describing clinical healthcare in SNOMED, laboratory tests in the LOINC, and diseases in the ICD-9.

The panelists further noted that determining which data elements should be included in an adverse medical event report may be easier than might first be expected, in part because there is already considerable agreement on what those elements should be. This view is supported by our examination of the 23 currently existing statewide reporting systems, which revealed that, while there are indeed differences across these systems, there is also considerable overlap, both in terms of the kinds of adverse medical events reported and the information gathered about these events. For example, 16 of the current state tracking systems collect information on surgical events; of these, 15 distinguish among surgical events that involve the wrong site, wrong patient, and/or wrong procedure. Nine of the state systems also, in some manner, ask about faulty instrument counts that result in foreign objects being left in surgical patients. The pattern is similar for all other information collected about adverse medical events by the patient safety tracking systems of the 23 states. In short, the differences among the existing, statewide adverse medical event reporting systems appear to be bridgeable, assuming that all parties are willing to give a little ground in an effort to achieve a common reporting system.

While the panelists noted that the advantages of standardizing adverse medical event reporting systems are apparent to virtually everyone involved with the healthcare industry, they conceded that precisely how to develop such standards and get all parties to incorporate the standards into their systems is not. Specifically, panelists noted that current efforts to develop standards on what to report to adverse medical event reporting systems are focused on standardizing the nomenclature for describing specific categories of adverse medical events, such as nosocomial infections and surgical incidents, rather than on standardizing the specific data elements that would comprise the ideal state patient safety tracking system. Others noted that one of the most ambitious standardization efforts currently under way—the HL7 effort to create standards for the exchange, management, and integration of electronic healthcare information—is focused on *how* information is to be shared, rather than on *what* information to share.

It was clear to panelists, however, that standardizing the vocabulary and grammar used to communicate patient information, laboratory tests, and other factors, as HL7 does, facilitates efforts to standardize the information transmitted to adverse medical event reporting systems. Panelists agreed that the data elements contained in the ideal adverse medical event reporting system should be viewed by states as the "minimum data set," which they can either adopt as a stand-alone system or use as the basis for a more encompassing patient safety tracking system.

MANAGING ADVERSE MEDICAL EVENT REPORTING SYSTEMS

While discussing what categories of information should be obtained about adverse medical events, several panelists noted that the front-line responsibility for actually reporting and/or recording the details about adverse medical events commonly falls on the shoulders of healthcare personnel who have limited training, both medical and otherwise. Consequently, while these healthcare workers may strive to diligently report the details of what appear to them to be serious adverse events, they may not possess the knowledge required to do so correctly. In short, concluding that a patient-harming adverse event has occurred often requires interpreting complex medical data that is beyond the analytic expertise of many healthcare professionals.

To deal with this problem, panelists suggested that, whenever possible, state adverse medical event reporting systems use predetermined menus (i.e., picklists) to help those reporting an adverse medical event provide all of the essential details to the system using the correct terminology. Panelists also suggested that, to the extent possible, consideration be given to developing and using a set of "global triggers" (i.e., flags) that, whenever they appear in patient charts and/or administrative records, will automatically prompt a review of all the relevant records by healthcare personnel who are qualified to determine whether a serious adverse medical event occurred. Such an approach to improving patient safety, particularly in the area of medications, has been recommended by the Institute for Healthcare Improvement in its work on the "Trigger Tool for Measuring Adverse Drug Events" (see Rozich, Haraden, and Resar, 2003).

Since adverse medical events, by their very nature, fall outside the realm of what is "routine" and/or "acceptable" at healthcare facilities, those who report such events would most likely want to be able to do so as easily as possible and without drawing undue attention to themselves. Consequently, the panelists thought that, although

consistency in the information reported is needed, it might be
counterproductive to dictate the form in which information about adverse
medical events is to be provided to a reporting system. Instead,
according to some panelists, the state system should be designed to
receive information on adverse medical events via mail, fax, and Web,
depending on the preferences of the reporter. The panelists did not
acknowledge that there is a trend among state reporting systems to move
towards 100 percent Web-based systems, and it is not clear how the idea
of an unconstrained reporting format might be implemented in a system
intended to provide uniformity in and accessibility to event reports.

The panelists noted, however, that the Web should clearly be used
by healthcare facilities to alert reporting parties to the need to
include specific pieces of information in their reports, regardless of
whether the report is ultimately submitted to the state reporting system
via Web, fax, or mail. The Web was also viewed by the panelists as a
useful means of informing healthcare workers about the ground rules
recommended by the panel for such reports. The panelists also
emphasized that employees must be assured that the information they
provide will be handled confidentially at the individual report level.
In short, it should be made clear to all healthcare personnel that
providing information to adverse medical event reporting systems is the
norm, not the exception, whenever adverse events that involve patients
occur.

Panelists noted, however, that healthcare facilities should audit
patient records, rather than relying entirely on incident reports to
obtain information on adverse medical events. That is, healthcare
facilities should maintain their patient records in a manner that
permits them to be reviewed regularly to identify anomalous events,
which can then be further investigated to determine whether a serious
adverse medical event has indeed occurred. The need for all healthcare
facilities to have such an audit capability was cited by panelists as
yet another reason why adverse medical event reporting systems need to
be standardized both within and across states. The panelists did not
address what role, if any, state authorities that oversee reporting
systems might play in such auditing.

Panelists agreed that it is important that the information collected in state adverse medical event reporting systems be assembled (via a parallel system) by a central entity that is both neutral and independent—something akin to the National Transportation Safety Board (NTSB), an independent federal agency charged with investigating every civil aviation accident in the United States—and that the information be made available to researchers, healthcare administrators, and policymakers. As noted in the first chapter of this report, by enacting the *Patient Safety and Quality Improvement Act of 2005*, the federal government has, indeed, begun to address the panelists' concerns about neutrality and independence in the collection and analysis of data regarding adverse medical events, albeit in a form quite different from that of the NTSB. Instead of establishing a body with responsibility for investigating adverse events, as NTSB does, the new law provides for the establishment of organizations—the PSOs—that will serve as a sort of data clearinghouse with an analytic capability. These organizations, which are the central feature of this new law, must themselves be neutral, independent entities. They are expressly prohibited from being health insurance issuers or components thereof and cannot be a part of any entity whose mission creates a conflict of interest with that of the PSO. In addition, any PSO that is a part of another entity must erect and maintain an impenetrable "firewall" between the PSO and the rest of the entity to prevent the sharing of any information. And the information provided by these PSOs to the network of databases created by the new law is to be made available to researchers, healthcare administrators, and policymakers. These features of the new law are thus compatible with the panel's emphasis on creating organizations to store and analyze patient safety that are likely to be perceived as impartial by the various actors involved in the healthcare system—both individual and institutional—and by the public.

SUMMARY

In a Web conference sponsored by RAND in April 2005, experts from a variety of disciplinary and institutional perspectives agreed that formal state-level adverse event reporting systems for reporting adverse medical events should be designed to capture information about events that cause harm to patients rather than information about all conceivable medical errors. They also agreed that efforts to create categorization schemes that can be used to describe adverse medical outcomes—for example, the list of never events specified by NQF—are positive developments and that states should rely on such already developed schemes in formulating and implementing their own reporting systems. The use of a common approach for categorizing adverse medical events will enable comparisons of the kinds and rates of such events across healthcare organizations and across geographic areas. The Web conference participants also agreed that institutional responsibility for collecting, storing, and disseminating information about adverse medical events must rest in neutral, independent organizations. They noted, however, that there are many practical obstacles to be overcome in developing and implementing state-level standards. The panelists did not address how to reconcile such institutional responsibilities with state responsibilities to follow up serious adverse events that cause harm.

8. SUMMARY AND CONCLUSIONS

This report summarizes three analytic efforts:

- A survey of state adverse medical event reporting systems
- An examination of the feasibility of using existing standards for reporting health information to characterize adverse medical events when they are recorded in formal event reporting systems
- A panel discussion focused on identifying properties of adverse event reporting systems that would permit comparative analyses by healthcare organizations, regulatory and accrediting organizations, and healthcare researchers and would embody characteristics to facilitate implementation and promote compliance.

Below we summarize our findings with regard to each of these topics.

FINDINGS: SURVEY OF STATE ADVERSE MEDICAL EVENT REPORTING SYSTEMS

Our survey examined both the administrative aspects of adverse medical event reporting systems (i.e., how data are collected and stored) and their content (i.e., what sorts of events are reported and what data elements are included in those reports).

Our findings indicate that 24 states have at least one formal adverse medical event reporting system, of which 20 are mandatory. Almost all of these systems required that hospitals submit reports of adverse events. General and acute care hospitals were cited most frequently as the kinds of facilities required to report adverse medical events, followed by ambulatory surgical centers, skilled nursing facilities, and psychiatric hospitals.

Most states require reporting of each reportable event; only two states require submission of aggregate counts of events. Most states require facilities to submit their reports using a statewide standard reporting form, but most allow multiple modes of submission—usually fax or mail. There is, however, a movement toward using Web-based systems as a means of submitting reports. Once submitted, reports of adverse events are stored in an electronic format of some sort, although in at least one state this meant that reports were saved as PDF files. The availability of electronic files, of course, facilitates analyses of adverse medical events across time, institutions, and states.

To be useful to researchers and policymakers seeking information about trends and patterns in the occurrence of adverse medical events, adverse medical event reporting systems must be well documented. Our research revealed, however, that in many instances such documentation (e.g., data dictionary, codebook, and entity relationship diagrams) is lacking. Only a few states were able to readily provide documentation about their electronically stored data and there is little agreement about what constitutes a data dictionary and codebook. Several states have recently established independent or semi-independent agencies to house adverse medical event reporting systems. Given their explicit focus on this activity, these agencies may be better able to keep the detailed records and documentation needed to pursue investigations of reporting patterns and patient safety outcomes, but, depending on how they are constituted, that advantage may be offset by privity of contract concerns involving the vendors that serve the agencies.

In terms of the content of reporting systems, we found that, since the release of the IOM report *To Err Is Human* (IOM 2000), consistency across state reporting systems has increased, in large part because, in defining adverse medical events, many states have relied on the list of 27 "never events" developed by NQF, the JCAHO list of sentinel events, or a combination of the two. In particular, since 2002, the number of states that require reporting of an NQF never event increased for 23 of the 27 never events.

The most commonly included NQF never events are
- patient death or serious disability associated with a medication error
- wrong-site surgery
- infant discharge to wrong person
- wrong-patient surgery
- wrong-procedure surgery

- retention of a foreign object.

The most commonly included JCAHO reviewable sentinel events are
- surgery performed on wrong patient or wrong body part
- hemolytic transfusion reaction
- rape.

After a description of the reportable event itself, the elements most commonly collected by state systems are a narrative of the event, information on corrective actions taken, when the event occurred, and patient information. Almost no national standard coding methods are used by states to collect information about adverse events.

ASSESSMENT OF THE UTILITY OF EXISTING MEDICAL STANDARDS FOR CODING ADVERSE MEDICAL EVENTS

A system for recording information regarding adverse medical events requires a coding system to capture information regarding the kind of event, where and when it occurred, who was involved, and so on. Thus, we attempted to determine whether existing health information standards could be applied to each of the IOM-recommended data elements for adverse medical event reporting. We based our assessment on a review of the 27 standards identified by the Consolidated Health Informatics (CHI) initiative, which is an effort directed by the U.S. Office of Management and the Budget to identify a portfolio of interoperability standards for health information. Our analysis suggests that efforts to develop standards for reporting adverse medical events can build on the CHI standards. Many of the detailed standards already exist for particular data elements, such as patient and product information. Thus, it should not be necessary to develop special standards for coding information about adverse medical events; such standards already exist or are being developed within the existing framework of other standardization efforts.

PROMULGATING NATIONAL PATIENT SAFETY STANDARDS

As part of our investigation, we convened an expert panel to discuss issues involved in developing and implementing a national adverse event reporting system. Panel members generally agreed that such a system should be simple, focused on adverse events that cause harm to patients (as opposed to capturing all medical errors), and administered by an organization that is not part of an entity that either provides or pays for healthcare. This last provision is important because, the panelists argued, ensuring the independence of a patient safety data collection and management organization would be essential to obtaining the cooperation of healthcare organizations and personnel.

A number of suggestions concerning the implementation of adverse medical event reporting systems were also offered. Perhaps the most important of these was that the skills of the people who would actually carry out the reporting need to be taken into account; doing so might mean, for instance, that reporting systems use predetermined menus to ensure that all the essential details are reported using the correct terminology. The panelists also emphasized that employees must be assured that the information they provide will be handled confidentially and that the information will be used primarily to improve institutional practices. They noted, too, that rather than relying solely on incident reports to obtain information on adverse medical events, healthcare facilities should also audit patient records regularly to identify anomalous events.

RECOMMENDATIONS FOR ESTABLISHING A NATIONAL REPOSITORY OF PATIENT SAFETY INFORMATION

Our analysis of current adverse reporting systems, existing procedures for coding information related to health and healthcare, and the views offered by our panelists lead to the recommendations below, which we believe will provide useful direction in the event that AHRQ moves to establish a national repository of state-provided standard patient safety information.

- **Create and maintain a database containing the information needed to track system characteristics over time.**

  Such a database should contain information concerning characteristics of the system, including the date it was implemented, when it was last modified, names of informants, their titles, and contact information.

- **Provide guidance to states regarding the supporting documentation for adverse event reporting systems.**
  To facilitate coordination and comparison across states, system characteristics and requirements must be documented. The federal government or another entity with experience in creating such documentation will likely need to provide guidance to states as to the types and formats of the materials needed and the format in which the data should be reported. In addition, as states move toward Web-based systems, additional guidance may be needed to develop database documentation that captures the characteristics of an electronic system.

- **In future research, determine how variations in definitions of reportable events affect cross-state comparisons of patient safety outcomes.**
  Many comparisons, and related validity studies, are needed to determine how particular variations in definitions of reportable events affect the assessment of patient safety outcomes. For example, researchers might compare adverse event rates under F system that requires reporting an event only if it results in severe patient injury or death with the rates under a system that requires the reporting of any incident regardless of patient harm. Given the variety of ways in which event definitions might differ, considerable research will be needed to settle on a set of definitions that can be used to reliably capture patient safety outcomes.

FINAL OBSERVATIONS

Although the *Patient Safety and Quality Improvement Act of 2005*, discussed in both Chapter 1 and Chapter 7, may increase the likelihood that states and healthcare systems will focus on the development and implementation of adverse medical event reporting systems, we believe that a national adverse event reporting system with "teeth" will require federal guidance. Even if mandatory state-level reporting systems are implemented, it is unlikely that the states will achieve the level of uniformity in their adverse medical event reporting systems required to monitor the occurrence of such events nationally without such guidance.

The federal government could facilitate such a system by sponsoring workshops to help the states develop a common set of standards for tracking the safety of patients in healthcare facilities. The government could also give grants to cover the costs of implementing these standards. To reinforce the importance of maintaining these systems, the federal government, in collaboration with the states, could amend the Medicare claims processes to require that all healthcare facilities receiving payments from CMS and having the agreed-upon patient safety systems in place receive bonus payments. Concomitantly, a dedicated unit within AHRQ could be established to assemble, analyze, and report on the information provided to patient safety tracking systems of all the states. This approach to standardizing the patient safety tracking systems across the nation will undoubtedly take some time to accomplish, but collaborating with the states in this effort should help to ensure that all states buy into it.

There are two alternatives to a state-federal collaborative model. The first—federal inaction and autonomous action by individual states—will only produce newer versions of the varying outcomes documented in this report. States will adopt and adapt guidelines being promulgated by various entities, such as NQF and JCAHO, or they will adopt their own idiosyncratic list. There will be considerable variation in how information is collected, transmitted, and stored, thereby making it nearly impossible to develop a national repository of patient safety reports that could be used as a basis for monitoring progress and formulating policy.

The second alternative is direct federal intervention and control. This approach would require establishing yet another reporting system beyond those currently required by the states, the risk management systems implemented by individual institutions, and any other systems that facilities may be required to participate in. In addition to imposing additional burdens on facilities (and thereby risking their support for such a system), direct federal intervention would be more costly and less efficient than collaborating with states. The results of our survey show that states have been quick to adopt or adapt reporting systems that incorporate recommendations made in *To Err Is Human* (IOM, 2001), suggesting that federal directives may not be necessary. It is possible, however, that states that have not yet modified their systems may be unwilling to do so in the absence of federal intervention.

APPENDIX

A.   CREATING ANALYTIC FILES OR WORKSHEETS

Using the information we obtained in the state surveys, we created a set of worksheets. Each worksheet corresponded to one of the 19 elements recommended by the IOM (see Table 2.2), with an additional "catchall" sheet that includes any elements not captured in the set of IOM recommendations. For each element, all unique "levels" or categories were entered in the rows of the worksheet. For example, reportable event is considered an element. If a state had 27 reportable events, each event was entered in the worksheet as a separate row or level.

When entering these elements, we retained the precise wording used by the state. For instance, if a state asked for "age" and another state asked "age in years," then "age" is entered and "age in years" is entered separately to retain the unique wording. Within each domain, we grouped like with like. For domains in which there were many variations in the wording of elements that were of central interest to this report (e.g., "what happened—event type"), we created subcategories to better represent the broad classes of event types while preserving the specific wording.

The columns correspond to each state with a reporting system. Only if the wording of a question was exactly the same do two or more states have the same level within an element. Because the exact wording often varied when going from the reporting forms to the description of the system to the authorizing law (or executive order creating the system), we decided to use the description of levels provided on the reporting forms first, followed by the system description, followed by law (if none of the prior were made available or existed). One member of the project team entered the information into the spreadsheet, and a second member verified the categorization.

Once a worksheet was verified, we organized or grouped the entries into categories. For example, all rows on the reportable event spreadsheet that corresponded to surgical events were grouped together. When appropriate, we did further groupings into subcategories. This allowed us to draw summary conclusions about the extent of consistency and inconsistency across states in how they report events. These analytic worksheets will be provided to AHRQ under separate cover.

**B. SUMMARY OF INFORMATION COLLECTED ABOUT EACH STATE SYSTEM
(INCLUDING MARYLAND)**

This table summarizes information that we collected as part of the 50-state survey that is not described elsewhere in the report.

Table B.1. Additional Descriptive Information from State-Level Survey

State	CALIFORNIA
System name	ACCLAIMS
Organization	California Department of Health Services
Detail on recoding	No recoding
State	**COLORADO**
System name	Occurrence Reporting Program
Organization	Department of Public Health and Environment
Detail on recoding	None
Other information	http://www.cdphe.state.co.us/hf/static/ncfocc.htm Reporting Manual, Note to customers and reporting forms for providers
State	**CONNECTICUT**
System name	Adverse Event Reporting
Organization	Department of Public Health
Detail on recoding	None
Other information	Reporting form and instructions: http://www.dph.state.ct.us/BHCS/AEreporting.htm
State	**FLORIDA**
System name	Healthcare Risk Management
Organization	State of Florida, Agency for Health Care Administration, Division of Health Quality Assurance
Detail on recoding	None provided.
Other information	For additional background information, see: http://www.fdhc.state.fl.us/MCHQ/Health_Facility_Regulation/Risk/reporting.shtml
State	**GEORGIA**
System name	Event Reporting System
Organization	Partnership for a Health and Accountability (PHA)
Detail on recoding	None
State	**KANSAS**
System name	Risk Management
Organization	Department of Health and Environment
Definition of reportable event	Reportable if determined to be so by facility's Risk Management committee
Detail on recoding	None

Other information	Quarterly report form: http://www.kdheks.gov/bhfr/download/quarterly_report_for m_rm_instructions.pdf
State	**MAINE**
System name	Sentinel Event Reporting
Organization	Maine Department of Health & Human Services, Division of Licensing and Certification
Detail on recoding	None
Other information	Sentinel Event Reporting Form available at: http://www.maine.gov/bms/providerfiles/sentinel_reportin g_forms.htm (last accessed July 13, 2006)
State	**MARYLAND**
System name	Maryland Patient Safety Program
Organization	Maryland Department of Health and Mental Hygiene, Office of Health Care Quality
Mandatory/voluntary	Mandatory
Aggregate/incident	Incident reports
Patient safety orientation	Yes
Year implemented	2004
Standard reporting form required?	No.
Facilities that report	Hospitals
Submission method	Phone, fax, e-mail
System computerized	Yes
Detail on recoding	Missing information
State	**MASSACHUSETTS**
System name	Hospital Reporting of Serious Incidents
Organization	Department of Public Health
Detail on recoding	None.
Other information	http://www.mass.gov/dph/dhcq/cicletter/cir1298.htm http://www.mass.gov/dph/dhcq/cicletter/cir_letter_040343 9.htm
State	**MINNESOTA**
System name	Adverse Health Events Reporting Law http://www.health.state.mn.us/patientsafety/
Organization	Now Minnesota Hospital Association Full implementation starting 12/04: will be Minnesota Department of Health
Detail on recoding	No recoding of information that is provided.
Other information	Briefing on system available at: http://www.health.state.mn.us/patientsafety/lawoverview. pdf Description of reportable events: http://www.health.state.mn.us/patientsafety/adverse27eve nts.html

State	MISSISSIPPI
Organization	Health Facilities Licensure and Certification, Mississippi Department of Health
Detail on recoding	None.
State	**NEVADA**
System name	Nevada Sentinel Events Registry
Organization	Nevada State Health Division, Bureau of Health Planning and Statistics
Detail on recoding	No recoding of data.
Other information	Description of system and background: www.nvha.net.news/sentinelevents.ppt http://health2k.state.nv.us/sentinel/
State	**NEW JERSEY**
System name	Patient Safety Act (passed in 2004) http://www.state.nj.us/health/hcqo/ps/legislation.shtml
Organization	Health Care Quality Assessment, Division of Health Care Quality and Oversight, Department of Health and Human Services
Detail on recoding	To be determined in consultation with vendor (to be selected).
Other information	2004 bill: http://www.njleg.state.nj.us/2004/Bills/S1000/557_R1.HTM
State	**NEW YORK**
System name	New York Patient Occurrence and Tracking System (NYPORTS)
Organization	Bureau of Hospital and Primary Care Services, Office of Health Systems Management, New York State Department of Health
Detail on recoding	None provided.
State	**PENNSYLVANIA**
System name	PA-PSRS (Pennsylvania Patient Safety Reporting System)
Organization	Patient Safety Authority
Detail on recoding	Definite recoding and reanalysis.
Other information	Act establishing the PSA: http://www.psa.state.pa.us/psa/lib/psa/act_13/act_13.pdf
State	**RHODE ISLAND**
System name	Rhode Island Hospital Incident and Event Reporting
Organization	Rhode Island Department of Health
Detail on recoding	None. Reports are returned to DOH, DOH reads them and decided to investigate or not. Report is filed away.
Other information	Section 34 of http://www.rules.state.ri.us/rules/released/pdf/DOH/DOH_3079.pdf Original law http://www.rilin.state.ri.us/Statutes/TITLE23/23-17/23-17-40.HTM

	In 2001, Dept. of Health received funding to review and analyze old reports and produced report available at this link: http://www.health.ri.gov/hsr/facilities/hospitals/hospitals2001.pdf. No funding has been available since then to update this analysis.
State	**SOUTH CAROLINA**
Organization	Department of Health and Environmental Control
Information requested	See definition of reportable event above.
Detail on recoding	None.
State	**TENNESSEE**
System name	Unusual Incident Reporting System
Organization	Tennessee Department of Public Health
Detail on recoding	None at this time.
Other information	See http://170.142.107.162/forms/G4010185cap.pdf for interpretative guidelines for all definitions. http://www2.state.tn.us/health/IPS/68-11-211.pdf
State	**TEXAS**
System name	Patient Safety Program and Medical Error Reporting
Organization	Department of Health
Detail on recoding	None
Other information	Patient Safety URL http://www.dshs.state.tx.us/hfp/default.shtm
State	**UTAH**
System name	Patient Safety Sentinel Event Reporting
Organization	Utah Department of Health
Detail on recoding	None.
Other information	Link to system: http://health.utah.gov/psi/.
State	**WASHINGTON**
System name	Rules 145 (10)
Organization	Washington State Department of Health
Detail on recoding	None.
Other information	www.doh.wa.gov/hsqa/fsl/hhhacs_hospitals.htm
State	**WYOMING**
System name	Wyoming Adverse Event Reporting System
Organization	Office of Health Facilities, Department of Health
Detail on recoding	None

C. HIERARCHICAL CATEGORIZATION OF REPORTABLE ADVERSE EVENTS

The tables below show the grouping of reportable adverse events in 14 states down to three levels of aggregation. Table C-1 shows the hierarchical categorization down to Level 2 and Level 3, respectively, where Level 1 is the most general grouping and Level 3 is the most detailed. Table C-2 shows the organization down to Level 4 (i.e., the wording of the specific events). An "R" indicates that a state requires that facilities report the defined event. Numbers above "R" indicate the hierarchy level of the category of reportable events into which the definition falls.

Table C.1. Hierarchical Categorization of Reportable Adverse Events, Levels 1, 2, and 3

Level 1	Level 2	Level 3		
1 0 0 0				SURGICAL EVENTS
	1 1 0 0			WRONG SITE/PATIENT/PROCEDURE
		1 1 1 0		WRONG SITE
		1 1 2 0		WRONG PATIENT
		1 1 3 0		WRONG PROCEDURE
		1 1 4 0		VARIOUS COMBINATIONS OF THE ABOVE
	1 2 0 0			FOREIGN OBJECT IN PATIENT/INCORRECT COUNT
		1 2 1 0		FOREIGN OBJECT LEFT IN PATIENT
		1 2 2 0		INCOMPLETE COUNT/COUNT NOT PERFORMED
		1 2 3 0		VARIOUS COMBINATIONS OF THE ABOVE
	1 3 0 0			VARIOUS COMBINATIONS OF THE ABOVE
	1 4 0 0			DEATH DURING OR IMMEDIATELY AFTER PROCEDURE
	1 5 0 0			COMPLICATION FOLLOWING PROCEDURE
		1 5 1 0		UNPLANNED SURGICAL PROCEDURE
		1 5 2 0		WOUND DEHISCENCE/INFECTION
		1 5 3 0		THROMBOSIS
		1 5 4 0		PULMONARY EMBOLISM
		1 5 5 0		PNEUMOTHORAX
		1 5 6 0		NEUROLOGICAL DEFICIT
		1 5 7 0		OTHER
	1 6 0 0			ERROR RELATED TO PROCEDURE
	1 7 0 0			OTHER
2 0 0 0				PRODUCT OR DEVICE EVENTS
	2 1 0 0			CONTAMINATED DRUGS, DEVICES, OR BIOLOGICS
	2 2 0 0			EQUIPMENT/DEVICE USE OR SAFETY PROBLEMS
		2 2 1 0		MALFUNCTION
		2 2 2 0		MISUSE
		2 2 3 0		OTHER
	2 3 0 0			DEVICE USED OR FUNCTIONS OTHER THAN AS INTENDED
	2 4 0 0			VARIOUS COMBINATIONS
	2 5 0 0			INTRAVASCULAR AIR EMBOLISM
	2 6 0 0			OTHER
3 0 0 0				PATIENT PROTECTION
	3 1 0 0			WRONG DISCHARGE
	3 2 0 0			ELOPEMENT
		3 2 1 0		DEATH OR OTHER INJURY
		3 2 2 0		MISSING PATIENT
	3 3 0 0			SELF-HARM

- 109 -

Level 1	Level 2	Level 3			

				Description
3	3	1	0	SUICIDE
3	3	2	0	ATTEMPTED SUICIDE/SELF-HARM
3	3	3	0	COMBINATION SUICIDE/ATTEMPTED SUICIDE
3	4	0	0	OTHER
4	**0**	**0**	**0**	**CARE MANAGEMENT**
4	1	0	0	MEDICATION ERRORS
4	1	1	0	SERIOUS OUTCOMES
4	1	2	0	DOSAGE ERROR
4	1	3	0	OTHER DRUG ADMINISTRATION ERRORS
4	1	4	0	ADVERSE DRUG REACTION
4	1	5	0	MONITORING ERROR
4	1	6	0	OTHER
4	2	0	0	TRANSFUSION EVENTS
4	2	1	0	SERIOUS OUTCOMES
4	2	2	0	REACTIONS
4	2	3	0	BLOOD TRANSFUSION ERRORS
4	2	4	0	OTHER
4	3	0	0	MATERNAL COMPLICATIONS
4	3	1	0	MATERNAL DEATH OR OTHER SERIOUS OUTCOME
4	3	2	0	FETAL DEATH OR OTHER SERIOUS OUTCOME
4	3	3	0	OTHER COMPLICATION
4	4	0	0	HYPOGLYCEMIA
4	5	0	0	HYPERBILIRUBINEMIA
4	6	0	0	ULCERS
4	7	0	0	SPINAL MANIPULATIVE THERAPY
4	8	0	0	SERIOUS PATIENT OUTCOMES DUE TO OTHER CARE MANAGEMENT ERRORS
4	8	1	0	GENERAL DEATHS
4	8	2	0	DEATH OR SERIOUS OUTCOMES ATTRIBUTED TO TREATMENT PROBLEM
4	8	3	0	PHYSICAL IMPAIRMENT
4	8	4	0	MENTAL IMPAIRMENT/BRAIN INJURY
4	8	5	0	SPINAL CORD INJURY
4	8	6	0	COMBINATION OF OUTCOMES
4	8	7	0	OTHER COMPLICATIONS
4	9	0	0	NOSOCOMIAL INFECTIONS
4	10	0	0	ANESTHESIA EVENT
4	11	0	0	RESPIRATORY CARE
4	12	0	0	OTHER COMPLICATIONS
4	12	1	0	EXTENDED HOSPITAL STAY/TRANSFERS
4	12	2	0	UNPLANNED PROCEDURES
4	12	3	0	EMERGENCY DEPARTMENT EVENT
4	12	4	0	LABORATORY TEST PROBLEMS
4	12	5	0	OTHER
4	13	0	0	RADIOLOGY/IMAGING PROBLEMS

Level 1	Level 2	Level 3		
		4	13 1 0	REFERRAL/CONSULT PROBLEM
4	14	0 0		NEGLECT
4	15	0 0		OTHER
4	16	0 0		COMBINATION OF ABOVE

5 0 0 0	ENVIRONMENTAL EVENTS

Level 1	Level 2	Level 3		
5	1	0 0		ELECTRIC SHOCK
5	2	0 0		WRONG OR CONTAMINATED GAS/SUBSTANCES
5	3	0 0		SKIN INTEGRITY
		5	3 1 0	BURN
		5	3 2 0	OTHER
5	4	0 0		FALLS
		5	4 1 0	DEATH OR OTHER INJURY
		5	4 2 0	ACTIVITY/LOCATION OF FALL
5	5	0 0		RESTRAINTS/BEDRAILS
5	6	0 0		SERVICE DISRUPTION
		5	6 1 0	DUE TO ADVERSE CONDITIONS OR DISASTER
		5	6 2 0	TERMINATION OF SERVICES
		5	6 3 0	INTERRUPTION OF SERVICES
		5	6 4 0	OTHER
5	7	0 0		INFECTIOUS OUTBREAKS
5	8	0 0		STRIKES
5	9	0 0		EMERGENCY SITUATIONS/DISASTERS
5	10	0 0		POISONING
5	11	0 0		FIRE
5	12	0 0		ADMINISTRATION AND MANAGEMENT PROBLEMS
5	13	0 0		COMBINATION OF ABOVE
5	14	0 0		OTHER

6 0 0 0	CRIMINAL EVENTS

Level 1	Level 2	Level 3	
6	1	0 0	IMPERSONATION OF HEALTH CARE PROVIDER
6	2	0 0	PATIENT ABDUCTION
6	3	0 0	SEXUAL ASSAULT
6	4	0 0	PHYSICAL ASSAULT
6	5	0 0	VERBAL OR UNSPECIFIED ASSAULT
6	6	0 0	SUSPICIOUS DEATH OR INJURY
6	7	0 0	MISAPPROPRIATION
6	8	0 0	OTHER POTENTIALLY CRIMINAL ACTIVITIES

Table C.2. Events Types Across 13 States (14 Systems) with Standard Report Forms, Nine States Without Standard Report Forms, JCAHO Sentinel Events, and NQF Serious Adverse Events

Shaded columns denote entries for the 14 systems with standard report forms.

Level 1	Level 2	Level 3	Level 4		CA	CO	CT	FL	GA-PHA	GA-GDHR	KS	ME	MN	MS	NV	NJ	NY	OR	PA	RI	SC	SD	TN	TX	UT	WA	WY	JCAHO	NQF
1	0	0	0	**SURGICAL EVENTS**																									
1	1	0	0	WRONG SITE/ PATIENT/PROCEDURE		1	1	1	1	1		1	1		1	1	1	1	1	1			1	1	1	1	1	1	1
1	1	1	0	WRONG SITE		2	2	2	2	2		2	2		2	2	2	2	2	2			2	2	2	2	2	2	2
1	1	1	1	Surgery performed on the wrong body part		3	3	3	3				3			3		3	3										3
1	1	1	2	Wrong body part		R		R					R			R		R	R										R
1	1	1	3	Surgical procedure performed on the wrong site																									
1	1	1	4	Wrong site																									
1	1	1	5	Wrong side (L vs. R)																									
1	1	2	0	WRONG PATIENT		3	3	3	3				3			3		3	3	3								3	3
1	1	2	1	Surgery performed on the wrong patient		R							R			R		R	R										R
1	1	2	2	Surgery on the wrong patient																									
1	1	2	3	Surgical procedure performed on the wrong patient				R											R	R									
1	1	2	4	Wrong patient																									
1	1	3	0	WRONG PROCEDURE		3	3	3	3				3			3		3	3									3	3
1	1	3	1	Wrong surgical procedure performed on a patient		R							R			R		R	R										R
1	1	3	2	Wrong surgical procedure performed				R											R										
1	1	3	3	ID missing/incorrect															R										
1	1	3	4	Surgical procedure unrelated to the patient's diagnosis				R					R			R			R										R
1	1	3	5	Wrong procedure																									
1	1	4	0	VARIOUS COMBINATIONS OF THE ABOVE				3	3			3			3	3	3		3				3	3	3	3	3	3	
1	1	4	1	Surgery performed on the wrong patient or wrong body part																						R		R	

Level 1	Level 2	Level 3	Level 4	#	Description	CA	CO	CT	FL	GA-PHA	GA-GDHR	KS	ME	MN	MS	NV	NJ	NY	OR	PA	RI	SC	SD	TN	TX	UT	WA	WY	JCAHO	NOF
1	1		4	2	Any surgery on the wrong patient or the wrong body part of the patient					R	R																			
1	1		4	3	A surgical procedure on the wrong patient or on the wrong body part of the patient																				R	R				
1	1		4	4	Surgery on the wrong patient or body part								R																	
1	1		4	5	Wrong Patient, Wrong Site - Surgical Procedure																			R						
1	1		4	6	Wrong Site/Surgery Procedure -- Actual Death											R		R												
1	1		4	7	Wrong Site/Surgery Procedure -- Actual Physical Injury with Permanent Loss											R														
1	1		4	8	Wrong Site/Surgery Procedure -- Actual Psychological Injury with Permanent Loss											R														
1	1		4	9	Wrong Site/Surgery Procedure -- Actual Physical and Psychological Injuries with Permanent Losses											R														
1	1		4	10	Wrong Site/Surgery Procedure -- Risk of Death											R														
1	1		4	11	Wrong Site/Surgery Procedure -- Risk of Physical Injury with Permanent Loss											R														
1	1		4	12	Wrong Site/Surgery Procedure -- Risk of Psychological Injury with Permanent Loss											R														
1	1		4	13	Wrong Patient/Wrong Surgery Procedure -- Actual Death											R														
1	1		4	14	Wrong Patient/Wrong Surgery Procedure -- Actual Physical Injury with Permanent Loss											R														
1	1		4	15	Wrong Patient/Wrong Surgery Procedure -- Actual Psychological Injury with Permanent Loss																									
1	1		4	16	Wrong Patient/Wrong Surgery Procedure -- Actual Physical and Psychological Injuries with Permanent Losses											R														
1	1		4	17	Wrong Patient/Wrong Surgery Procedure -- Risk of Death											R														
1	1		4	18	Wrong Patient/Wrong Surgery Procedure -- Risk of Physical Injury with Permanent Loss											R														
1	1		4	19	Wrong Patient/Wrong Surgery Procedure -- Risk of Psychological Injury with Permanent Loss											R														

Level 1	Level 2	Level 3	Level 4	Description	CA	CO	CT	FL	GA-PHA	GA-GDHR	KS	ME	MN	MS	NV	NJ	NY	OR	PA	RI	SC	SD	TN	TX	UT	WA	WY	JCAHO	NQF
1	2	0	0	FOREIGN OBJECT IN PATIENT/INCORRECT COUNT		3	2	2					2			2	2	2	2				2	2					2
	2	1	0	FOREIGN OBJECT LEFT IN PATIENT			3	3					3			3		3	3				3	3					3
	2	1	1	Retention of a foreign object in a patient after surgery or other procedure			R	R					R			R		R						R					R
	2	1	2	Foreign object retention																									
	2	1	3	A foreign object accidentally left in a patient during a procedure																									
	2	1	4	foreign objects remaining from a surgical procedure																									
	2	1	5	Foreign body in patient																									
	2	2	0	INCOMPLETE COUNT/ COUNT NOT PERFORMED																									
	2	2	1	Count incomplete/not performed															R										
	2	2	2	Count incorrect-needles															3										
	2	2	3	Count incorrect-sponges													3		R				3						
	2	2	4	Count incorrect-equipment															R										
	2	3	0	VARIOUS COMBINATIONS OF THE ABOVE — Unintentionally retained foreign body due to inaccurate surgical count or break in procedural													R		R										
	2	3	1	technique (sponges, lap pads, instruments, guidewires from central line insertion, cut intravascular cannulas, needles, etc.)																			R						
1	3	0	0	VARIOUS COMBINATIONS OF THE ABOVE					2																				
	3	0	1	Surgical event (includes wrong site surgery, surgery performed on wrong patient, wrong surgical procedure, retention of foreign object in patient, and post-operative death in an ASA Class I patient)					R																				2
1	4	0	0	DEATH DURING OR IMMEDIATELY AFTER PROCEDURE																									
	4	0	1	Intra/Post-Op Death		2	2						2			2	2	2											
	4	0	2	Intraoperative or immediate post-operative death in an ASA (American Society of Anesthesiology) Class I patient		R	R						R																

Level 1	Level 2	Level 3	Level 4	Description	CA	CO	CT	FL	GA-PHA	GA-GDHR	KS	ME	MN	MS	NV	NJ	NY	OR	PA	RI	SC	SD	TN	TX	UT	WA	WY	JCAHO	NQF
1	4	0	3	Intraoperative or immediately post-operative death in an ASA Class I patient																									
1	4	0	4	Intraoperative or immediately post-operative coma or death in an ASA Class I (hospital) or any ASA Class I patient (ambulatory surgery center)												R	R	R											R
1	4	0	5	Other event causing patient death or harm that lasts seven days or is present at discharge												R													
1	4	0	6	Death occurring after a specific procedure (ICD-9 47.0-47.19, 88.4-88.49, 51.2-51.24, 38.10-38.19, 45.7-45.8, 68.3-68.7, 68.9, 45.23-45.24, 60.2-60.69, 81.5-81.59, 81.0-81.09)																									
1	5	0	0	COMPLICATION FOLLOWING PROCEDURE				2									2		2				2						
1	5	1	0	UNPLANNED SURGICAL PROCEDURE				3											3										
1	5	1	1	Unplanned return to operating room													R		R										
1	5	1	2	Surgical repair of injuries from a planned surgical procedure				R																					
1	5	2	0	WOUND DEHISCENCE/INFECTION													3		3				3						
1	5	2	1	Wound dehiscence requiring repair													R		R										
1	5	2	2	Wound dehiscence																									
1	5	2	3	Post-op surgical wound infection, following clean or clean/contaminated case (Performed in the O.R. or Surgical suite only) requiring drainage during the hospital stay or inpatient hospital admission within 30 days													R		R										
1	5	2	4	Post-op wound infection following clean or clean/contaminated case																									
1	5	2	5	Necrosis or infection requiring repair (incision and drainage (I&D), debridement, or other surgical intervention), regardless of the location for the repair (e.g., at the bedside, in a treatment room, in the OR)													R		R				R						
1	5	2	6	Wound or surgical site infection																									
1	5	3	0	THROMBOSIS																									
1	5	3	1	Deep venous thrombosis													3		3										
1	5	3	2	New documented deep vein thrombosis (DVT) at any site													R		R				R						

Level 1	Level 2	Level 3	Level 4	Description	CA	CO	CT	FL	GA-PHA	GA-GDHR	KS	ME	MN	MS	NV	NJ	NY	OR	PA	RI	SC	SD	TN	TX	UT	WA	WV	JCAHO	NQF
1	5	4	3	3 Thrombosed distal bypass graft requiring repair													R		3										
				PULMONARY EMBOLISM																									
1	5	0	4	1 New, acute pulmonary embolism, confirmed, or suspected and treated													3		3				3						
1	5		4	2 Pulmonary embolism													R		R										
				PNEUMOTHORAX																									
1	5	0	5	1 Pneumothorax													3		3				3						
1	5		5	2 Pneumothorax, regardless of size or treatment (includes pneumothoraces resulting from a procedure performed through an intravascular catheter, e.g., temporary pacemaker insertion)															R										
				NEUROLOGICAL DEFICIT																									
1	5	0	6	1 Any new central neurological deficit (e.g., TIA, stroke, hypoxic/anoxic encephalopathy)													R						R						
1	5		6	2 Any new peripheral neurological deficit (e.g., palsy, paresis) with motor weakness													3		3				3						
				OTHER																									
1	5	0	7	1 Removal of tube or other medical device by patient													R		R										
1	5	7	2	2 Hemorrhage or hematoma requiring drainage, evacuation or other procedural intervention													R		R										
1	5	7		3 Hemorrhage or hematoma requiring drainage, evacuation or other procedural intervention or results in serious injury or death															R										
1	5	7		4 Anastomotic leakage requiring repair													R						R						
1	5	7		5 Acute renal failure																									
1	5	7		6 AMI (Acute Myocardial Infarction) - unrelated to a cardiac procedure.													R		R										
1	5	7		7 Cardiac arrest with successful resuscitation.													R		R										
1	5	7		8 Cardiopulmonary arrest															R										
1	5	7		9 Myocardial infarction															R										
1	5	7		10 Unplanned transfer to ICU															R										
1	5	7		11 Stroke or other neurologic deficit															R										
1	5	7		12 Death															R										

Level 1	Level 2	Level 3	Level 4	Description	CA	CO	CT	FL	GA-PHA	GA-GDHR	KS	ME	MN	MS	NV	NJ	NY	OR	PA	RI	SC	SD	TN	TX	UT	WA	WY	JCAHO	NQF
1	5	7	13	Other (specify)													2		R										
1	6	0		ERROR RELATED TO PROCEDURE																									
			1	Break in sterile technique															2										
			2	Consent missing/inadequate															R										
			3	Preparation inadequate/wrong															R										
			4	Procedure not ordered															R										
			5	Procedure cancelled or not performed															R										
			6	Procedure delayed															R										
			7	Procedure not completed															R										
			8	Unintended laceration or puncture															R										
			9	All unplanned conversions to an open procedure because of an injury and/or bleeding during the laparoscopic procedure															R										
1	7	0	0	OTHER													R		2										
			1	Surgical error		1	1		1				1			1	1	1	1				1	1					1
			2	Others surgery/invasive procedure problem (specify)		2							2			2		2	2					1					2
2	0	0	0	PRODUCT OR DEVICE EVENTS																									
2	1	0	0	CONTAMINATED DRUGS, DEVICES, OR BIOLOGICS													2		2										
			1	Patient death or serious disability associated with the use of contaminated drugs, devices, or biologics provided by the healthcare facility		R							R			R	R	R	R										R
			2	Contaminated (resulting in death or serious disability only)																									
			3	Patient death or serious physical injury associated with the use of contaminated drugs, devices, or biologics provided by the healthcare facility																									
			4	Patient death/harm due to the use of contaminated drugs/devices/biologics															R										
			5	Contaminated drug/biologic																									
2	2	0	0	EQUIPMENT/DEVICE USE OR SAFETY PROBLEMS													2		2										

Level 1 / Level 2	Level 3	Level 4		CA	CO	CT	FL	GA-PHA	GA-GDHR	KS	ME	MN	MS	NV	NJ	NY	OR	PA	RI	SC	SD	TN	TX	UT	WA	WY	JCAHO	NQF
	2 2 1 0		MALFUNCTION													3		3										
		2 2 1 1	Malfunction of equipment during treatment or diagnosis or a defective product which resulted in death or serious injury													R												
		2 2 1 2	Malfunction of equipment during treatment or diagnosis or a defective product which has a potential for adversely affecting patient or hospital personnel or resulting in a retained foreign object													R												
		2 2 1 3	Equipment malfunction															R										
		2 2 1 4	Electrical problem															R										
		2 2 1 5	Failed test of standard procedures															R										
	2 2 2 0		MISUSE															3										
		2 2 2 1	Automated dispensing machine problem															I										
		2 2 2 2	Disconnected															R										
		2 2 2 3	Equipment misuse															R										
	2 2 3 0		OTHER															3										
		2 2 3 1	Equipment not available															R										
		2 2 3 2	Equipment wrong or inadequate															R										
		2 2 3 3	Medical device problem															R										
		2 2 3 4	Inadequate supplies															R										
		2 2 3 5	Preventive maintenance inadequate/not performed															R										
		2 2 3 6	Other (equipment safety situation)															R										
2 3 0 0			DEVICE USED OR FUNCTIONS OTHER THAN AS INTENDED			2		2				2			2								2					2
		2 3 0 1	Patient death or serious disability associated with the use or function of a device in patient care that is used or functions other than as intended			R																						R
		2 3 0 2	A patient death or serious disability associated with the use of or function of a device designed for a patient that is used or functions other than as intended																				R					

L1	L2	L3	L4	Description	CA	CO	CT	FL	GA-PHA	GA-GDHR	KS	ME	MN	MS	NV	NJ	NY	OR	PA	RI	SC	SD	TN	TX	UT	WA	WY	JCAHO	NQF
2	4	3	0	Product or device event (includes death or serious disability associated with use of contaminated drugs, devices, or biologics, device misuse/malfunction, and air embolism)																									
2	4	3	0	Patient death/harm due to the use/function of a device in patient care in which the device is used/functions other than as intended																									
2	4	3	0	Malfunction (resulting in death or serious disability only)					R				R			R													
2	4	0	0	VARIOUS COMBINATIONS		2												2	2										
2	4	4	0	Malfunction or intentional or unintentional misuse of equipment AND adverse affects or potentially adverse affects AND occurred during treatment or diagnosis		R												R											
2	4	4	0	Patient death or serious physical injury associated with the use or function of a device in patient care in which the device is poorly designed, or is used in functions other than as intended																									
2	5	0	0	INTRAVASCULAR AIR EMBOLISM		2							2			2			2										2
2	5	0		Patient death or serious disability associated with intravascular air embolism that occurs while being cared for in a healthcare facility														R											
2	5	0		Air embolism (resulting in death or serious disability only)		R							R																
2	5	0		Patient death or serious physical injury associated with intravascular air embolism that occurs while being cared for in a healthcare facility																									R
2	5	0		Patient death/harm due to intravascular air embolism																									
2	5	0		Intravascular air embolism																			2						
2	6	0	0	OTHER												R		R	R										
2	6	0		Other (equipment/supplies/devices)												2	2		2										
2	6	0		Displacement, migration or breakage of an implant, device, graft, or drain, whether repaired, intentionally left in place or removed													R		R				R						

Level 1	Level 2	Level 3	Level 4	Description	CA	CO	CT	FL	GA-PHA	GA-GDHR	KS	ME	MN	MS	NV	NJ	NY	OR	PA	RI	SC	SD	TN	TX	UT	WA	WY	JCAHO	NQF
	2	6	0	Other event causing patient death or harm that lasts seven days or is present at discharge	1	1	1		1			1	1	1	1	R	1	1	1	1		1	1	1	1	1	1	1	1
3	0	0		**PATIENT PROTECTION**												1													
3	1	0	0	WRONG DISCHARGE		2	2					2	2		2	1	2	2	2	2		2	2	1	2	1	1	1	2
3	1	0	1	Infant discharge																									
3	1	0	2	Infant discharged to the wrong person																									
3	1	0	3	Infant discharged to wrong family		R	R						R			R	R	R	I				R		R					R
3	1	0	4	Discharge of an infant to the wrong family																									
3	1	0	5	Infant abduction or discharge to the wrong family								R																	
3	1	0	6	Discharge of patient to wrong family																									
3	2	0	0	ELOPEMENT	2	2	2						2		2	2	2	2	2	2		2	2						2
3	2	1	0	DEATH OR OTHER INJURY		3	3						3		3	3		3	3	2		3	2						3
3	2	1	1	Patient death/harm due to patient elopement																									
3	2	1	2	Patient death or serious disability associated with patient elopement (disappearance) for more than four hours			R									R													
3	2	1	3	Patient death or serious physical injury associated with patient elopement (disappearance) for more than four hours		R							R					R											R
3	2	1	4	Elopement (resulting in death or serious disability)									R																
3	2	1	5	Elopement -- Actual Death																									
3	2	1	6	Elopement -- Actual Physical Injury with Permanent Loss											R														
3	2	1	7	Elopement -- Actual Psychological Injury with Permanent Loss											R														
3	2	1	8	Psychological Injuries with Permanent Losses											R														
3	2	1	9	Elopement -- Risk of Death											R														
3	2	1	10	Elopement -- Risk of Physical Injury with Permanent Loss											R														
3	2	1	11	Elopement -- Risk of Psychological Injury with Permanent Loss											R														
3	2	2	0	MISSING PATIENT	3	3	3								3		3		3	3		3	3						

Level 1	Level 2	Level 3	Level 4	Description	CA	CO	CT	FL	GA-PHA	GA-GDHR	KS	ME	MN	MS	NV	NJ	NY	OR	PA	RI	SC	SD	TN	TX	UT	WA	WY	JCAHO	NQF
3	0	0																											
3	2	2	1	Kidnapping and inpatient psychiatric elopements and elopements by minors																									
3	2	2	2	Elopement from hospital resulting in death or serious injury																R			R						
3	2	2	3	Inpatient elopement/AWOL													R		I			R							
3	2	2	4	Missing patient		2	2					2	2	2	2	2	2		2	2			2	2	2	2	2	2	2
3	2	2	5	At risk and missing after search conducted OR missing more than eight hours, regardless of risk		3						3			3					3				3	3	3	3	3	
3	2	2	6	Disappearance or loss of a patient or inmate-patient	R	R																					R		
3	3	0	0	SELF-HARM																									
3	3	1	0	SUICIDE																									
3	3	1	1	Suicide of a patient during treatment or within 5 days of discharge from an inpatient or outpatient unit (if known)																									
3	3	1	2	A patient suicide while the patient was under care in the hospital																									
3	3	1	3	Death resulting from suicide		R																							
3	3	1	4	Suicide																							R		
3	3	1	5	Suicide -- Actual Death											R											R			
3	3	1	6	Suicide -- Actual Physical Injury with Permanent Loss											R														
3	3	1	7	Suicide -- Actual Psychological Injury with Permanent Loss											R														
3	3	1	8	Suicide -- Actual Physical and Psychological Injuries with Permanent Losses											R														
3	3	1	9	Suicide -- Risk of Death											R														
3	3	1	10	Suicide -- Risk of Physical Injury with Permanent Loss											R														
3	3	1	11	Suicide -- Risk of Psychological Injury with Permanent Loss											R														
3	3	1	12	Suicide of a patient																									
3	3	1	13	Suicide of a patient in a setting in which the patient receives around-the-clock care																					R			R	
3	3	1	14	The suicide of a patient in a setting in which the patient received care 24 hours a day																				R					

Level 1	Level 2	Level 3	Level 4	#	Event	CO	CT	FL	GA-PHA	GA-GDHR	KS	ME	MN	MS	NV	NJ	NY	OR	PA	RI	SC	SD	TN	TX	UT	WA	WY	JCAHO	NQF
		3	3	1	Suicide of a patient in a healthcare facility where the patient receives inpatient care (15)							R																	
		3	3	0	**ATTEMPTED SUICIDE/SELF-HARM**																								
		3	3	2	1 Suicide attempt																								
		3	3	2	2 Self-harm or injury																								
		3	3	0	**COMBINATION SUICIDE/ATTEMPTED SUICIDE**																								
		3	3	1	Patient suicide, or attempted suicide resulting in serious disability, while being cared for in a healthcare facility	3							3	3		3	3		3				3						3
		3	3	2	Suicide or attempted suicide resulting in serious disability	R			R				R	R		R	R		1				R					R	
		3	3	3	Patient suicide/attempted suicide														1										
		3	3	4	Suicides and attempted suicides related to an inpatient hospitalization, with serious injury				2							2	R						R						
		3	3	5	Suicides and attempted suicides related to an inpatient hospitalization, with serious injury				R																				
3	4	0			**OTHER**																								
		3	4	1	Patient Protection Event (includes infant discharge to wrong person, death or serious disability associated with patient elopement and patient suicide/attempted suicide)																								
		3	4	0	Any serious preventable adverse event which results in death or loss of a body part or disability or loss of bodily function lasting more than seven (7) days or present at discharge											R													
4	0	0			**CARE MANAGEMENT**																								
4	1	0			**MEDICATION ERRORS**	1	1	1	1	1	1	1	1	1	1	1	1	1	1	1	1	1	1	1	1	1	1	1	1
		4	1	1	**SERIOUS OUTCOMES**																								
		4	1	1	A medication error occurred that resulted in a patient death	2	2						2		2	2	2	2	2		2		2	2			2	2	2
		4	1	1	Significant medication reactions resulting in death or serious disability	3 / R	3						3		3	3	3 / R	3					3 / R	3		3	3	3	3

Level 1	Level 2	Level 3	Level 4	Description	NQF	JCAHO	WY	WA	UT	TX	TN	SD	SC	RI	PA	OR	NY	NJ	NV	MS	MN	ME	KS	GA-GDHR	GA-PHA	FL	CT	CO	CA
4	1	1	3	A medication error resulting in a patient's unanticipated death or major permanent loss of bodily function in circumstances unrelated to the natural course of the illness or underlying condition of the patient																									
4	1	1	4	Med error (resulting in death or serious disability only)						R											R								
4	1	1	5	Patient death or serious physical injury associated with a medication error (e.g., errors involving the wrong drug, wrong dose, wrong patient, wrong time, wrong rate, wrong preparation or wrong route of administration)												R													
4	1	1	6	Patient death or serious disability associated with a medication error (e.g., errors involving the wrong drug, wrong dose, wrong patient, wrong time, wrong rate, wrong preparation or wrong route of administration)	R																								
4	1	1	7	Patient death/harm due to a medication error			R																					R	
4	1	1	8	Medication error that results in significant injury or death														R											
4	1	1	9	Medication error																									
4	1	1	10	Medication Error(s) -- Actual Death															R										
4	1	1	11	Medication Error(s) -- Actual Physical Injury with Permanent Loss															R										
4	1	1	12	Medication Error(s) -- Actual Psychological Injury with Permanent Loss															R										
4	1	1	13	Medication Error(s) -- Actual Physical and Psychological Injuries with Permanent Losses															R										
4	1	1	14	Medication Error(s) -- Risk of Death															R										
4	1	1	15	Medication Error(s) -- Risk of Physical Injury with Permanent Loss															R										
4	1	1	16	Medication Error(s) -- Risk of Psychological Injury with Permanent Loss													R		R										
4	1	1	17	A medication error occurred that resulted in permanent patient harm																									
4	1	1	18	A medication error occurred that resulted in a near-death event (e.g., cardiac or respiratory arrest requiring BLS or ACLS)							R						R												

Level 1	Level 2	Level 3	Level 4	#	Description	CA	CO	CT	FL	GA-PHA	GA-GDHR	KS	ME	MN	MS	NV	NJ	NY	OR	PA	RI	SC	SD	TN	TX	UT	WA	WY	JCAHO	NQF
4	1	1	19		A medication error occurred that resulted in a near-death event (e.g., an aphylaxis, cardiac arrest)															3				R						
4	1	2	0		DOSAGE ERROR																			3						
4	1	2	1		Wrong dose															R				R						
4	1	2	2		Wrong dose/over dosage															R										
4	1	2	3		Wrong dose/under dosage															R										
4	1	2	4		Wrong duration															R										
4	1	2	5		Dose omission																									
4	1	2	6		Omission															R				R						
4	1	2	7		Extra dose															R										
4	1	2	8		Wrong dosage form																									
4	1	3	0		OTHER DRUG ADMINISTRATION ERRORS															3				3						
4	1	3	1		Wrong drug															R				R						
4	1	3	2		Wrong route															R				R						
4	1	3	3		Wrong rate (IV)															R										
4	1	3	4		Wrong strength/concentration															R										
4	1	3	5		Wrong dilutent/concentration/dosage form																			R						
4	1	3	6		Prescription/refill delayed															R										
4	1	3	7		Wrong technique															R										
4	1	3	8		Wrong time															R										
4	1	3	9		Wrong patient															R				R						
4	1	3	10		Administration after order discontinued/expired																			R						
4	1	3	11		Medication list incorrect															R				R						
4	1	3	12		Wrong frequency																									
4	1	4	0		ADVERSE DRUG REACTION															3				R						
4	1	4	1		Rash															R										
4	1	4	2		Hypotension															R										
4	1	4	3		Arrhythmia															R										
4	1	4	4		Hematologic problem															R										
4	1	4	5		Nephrotoxicity															R										

Level 1	Level 2	Level 3	Level 4	Description	CA	CO	CT	FL	GA-PHA	GA-GDHR	KS	ME	MN	MS	NV	NJ	NY	OR	PA	RI	SC	SD	TN	TX	UT	WA	WY	JCAHO	NQF
4	1	4	6	Dizziness															R										
4	1	4	7	Mental status change															R										
4	1	4	8	Other (specify)															R				3						
4	1	5	0	MONITORING ERROR															3										
4	1	5	1	Drug-drug interaction															R										
4	1	5	2	Drug-food/nutrient interaction															R										
4	1	5	3	Documented allergy															R										
4	1	5	4	Drug-disease interaction															R										
4	1	5	5	Clinical (lab value, vital sign)															R				R						
4	1	5	6	Deteriorated drug/biologic															R		3								
4	1	5	7	Other (specify)															R										
4	1	5	8	Monitoring error																	R								
4	1	6	0	OTHER															3										
4	1	6	1	Unauthorized drug															R										
4	1	6	2	Inadequate pain management															I										
4	1	6	3	Other (medication safety)															R										
4	1	6	4	Other (medication error)																									
4	1	6	5	Incidents resulting in death or serious injury, e.g., a broken limb																									
4	2	0	0	TRANSFUSION EVENTS		2	2					2	2		2	2		2	2	2			2	2		2		2	2
4	2	1	0	SERIOUS OUTCOMES		3	3						3		3	3		3	2				2	2				2	3
4	2	1	1	Patient death or serious disability associated with a hemolytic reaction due to the administration of ABO-incompatible blood or blood products		R																							
4	2	1	2	Patient death or serious physical injury associated with a hemolytic reaction due to the administration of ABO-incompatible blood or blood products																									
4	2	1	3	Patient death/harm due to a hemolytic reaction due to the administration of ABO-incompatible blood or blood products																									
4	2	1	4	Transfusion -- Actual Death											R	R		R											R

Level 1	Level 2	Level 3	Level 4	Description	CA	CO	CT	FL	GA-PHA	GA-GDHR	KS	ME	MN	MS	NV	NJ	NY	OR	PA	RI	SC	SD	TN	TX	UT	WA	WV	JCAHO	NQF
4	2	1	5	Transfusion -- Actual Physical Injury with Permanent Loss											R														
4	2	1	6	Transfusion -- Actual Psychological Injury with Permanent Loss											R														
4	2	1	7	Transfusion -- Actual Physical and Psychological Injuries with Permanent Losses											R														
4	2	1	8	Transfusion -- Risk of Death											R														
4	2	1	9	Transfusion -- Risk of Physical Injury with Permanent Loss											R														
4	2	1	10	Transfusion -- Risk of Psychological Injury with Permanent Loss																									
4	2	1	11	Errors or reaction from transfusion of blood or blood products AND life-threatening		R									R														
4	2	1	12	Wrong blood product (resulting in death or serious disability only)																									
4	2	2	0	REACTIONS								3	R						3				3	3		3		3	
4	2	2	1	Hemolytic transfusion reaction involving the administration of blood or blood products having major blood group incompatibilities																									
4	2	2	2	A hemolytic transfusion reaction involving administration of blood or blood products having major blood group incompatibilities								R														R		R	
4	2	2	3	A hemolytic transfusion reaction in a patient resulting from the administration of blood or blood products with major blood group incompatibilities															R					R					
4	2	2	4	Blood transfusion reactions related to wrong type of blood																			R						
4	2	2	5	Apparent transfusion reaction																									
4	2	3	0	BLOOD TRANSFUSION ERRORS																									
4	2	3	1	Blood transfusion error															3	3			3						
4	2	3	2	Blood transfusion related to outdated blood, wrong patient																3									
4	2	3	3	Wrong patient requested															R	R			R						
4	2	3	4	Wrong patient transfused															R										
4	2	3	5	Event related to blood product administration															R										

Level 1	Level 2	Level 3	Level 4	Description	NQF	JCAHO	WY	WA	UT	TX	TN	SD	SC	RI	PA	OR	NY	NJ	NV	MS	MN	ME	KS	GA-GDHR	GA-PHA	FL	CT	CO	CA
4	2	3	6	Event related to blood product dispensing or distribution											R														
4	2	3	7	Event related to blood sample collection											R														
4	2	3	8	Mismatched unit											R														
4	2	3	9	Wrong component requested											R														
4	2	3	10	Wrong component issued											R														
4	2	3	11	Special product need not requested											R														
4	2	3	12	Special product need not issued											3														
4	2	4	0	OTHER											R														
4	2	4	1	Other (transfusion related -- specify)																									
4	3	0	0	MATERNAL COMPLICATIONS	2	2				2	2			2	2	2	2	2	2		2					2			
4	3	1	0	MATERNAL DEATH OR OTHER SERIOUS OUTCOME	3										3	3		3	3		3						3		
4	3	1	1	Maternal death or serious disability associated with labor or delivery in a low-risk pregnancy while being cared for in a healthcare facility																									
4	3	1	2	Maternal labor (resulting in death or serious disability only)												R					R						R		
4	3	1	3	Maternal death or serious physical injury associated with labor or delivery in a low-risk pregnancy while being cared for in a healthcare facility														R											
4	3	1	4	Maternal death/harm due to labor/delivery in a low-risk pregnancy																									
4	3	1	5	Maternal Intrapartum -- Actual Death															R										
4	3	1	6	Maternal Intrapartum -- Actual Physical Injury with Permanent Loss															R										
4	3	1	7	Maternal Intrapartum -- Actual Psychological Injury with Permanent Loss															R										
4	3	1	8	Maternal Intrapartum -- Actual Physical and Psychological Injuries with Permanent Losses															R										
4	3	1	9	Maternal Intrapartum -- Risk of Death															R										
4	3	1	10	Maternal Intrapartum -- Risk of Physical Injury with Permanent Loss															R										

Level 1	Level 2	Level 3	Level 4	#	Description	NQF	JCAHO	WY	WA	UT	TX	TN	SD	SC	RI	PA	OR	NY	NJ	NV	MS	MN	ME	KS	GA-GDHR	GA-PHA	FL	CT	CO	CA
4	3	1	11		Maternal Intrapartum -- Risk of Psychological Injury with Permanent Loss											R				R										
4	3	1	12		Death																									
4	3	2	0		FETAL DEATH OR OTHER SERIOUS OUTCOME		3				3				3	3	3			3							3	3		
4	3	2	1		Fetal death																						R			
4	3	2	2		A perinatal death unrelated to a congenital condition in an infant with a birth weight greater than 2,500 grams						R																			
4	3	2	3		Infant Perinatal -- Actual Death															R										
4	3	2	4		Infant Perinatal -- Actual Physical Injury with Permanent Loss															R										
4	3	2	5		Infant Perinatal -- Actual Psychological Injury with Permanent Loss															R										
4	3	2	6		Infant Perinatal -- Actual Physical and Psychological Injuries with Permanent Losses															R										
4	3	2	7		Infant Perinatal -- Risk of Death															R										
4	3	2	8		Infant Perinatal -- Risk of Physical Injury with Permanent Loss											R				R										
4	3	2	9		Infant Perinatal -- Risk of Psychological Injury with Permanent Loss											R														
4	3	2	10		Any perinatal death or serious physical injury unrelated to a congenital condition in an infant having a birth weight greater than 2500 grams												R													
4	3	2	11		Intrapartum fetal death																									
4	3	2	12		Neonatal death																									
4	3	2	13		Obstetrical events resulting in death or serious disability to the neonate											R												R		
4	3	2	14		Birth injury or trauma											R														
4	3	2	15		Unanticipated death of a full-term infant																									
4	3	2	16		Any incidence resulting in birth injury not within normal range of patient outcomes		R								R	R														
4	3	2	17		Unplanned Transfer to NICU																									
4	3	0			OTHER COMPLICATION							3				3		3												

Level 1	Level 2	Level 3	Level 4	Description	CA	CO	CT	FL	GA-PHA	GA-GDHR	KS	ME	MN	MS	NV	NJ	NY	OR	PA	RI	SC	SD	TN	TX	UT	WA	WY	JCAHO	NQF
			4 3	1 Unplanned postpartum hysterectomy													R						R						
			4 3	2 Hysterectomy in a pregnant woman												R	R		R											
			4 3	3 Inverted uterus															R											
			4 3	4 Unplanned transfer to ICU															R											
			4 3	5 Ruptured uterus													R		R				R							
			4 3	6 Uterine rupture															R											
			4 3	7 Unanticipated blood transfusion															R											
			4 3	8 DVT (Deep Venous Thrombosis)															R											
			4 3	9 PE (pulmonary embolism)															R											
			4 3	10 Seizure													R		R				R							
			4 3	11 Infection															R											
			4 3	12 Apgar <5 at 5 min															R											
			4 3	13 Circumcision requiring repair															2											
			4 3	14 Other (specify)		2										2		2												2
4 4 0				**HYPOGLYCEMIA**																									
			4 4 0	1 Patient death/harm due to hypoglycemia																									
			4 4 0	2 Patient death or serious disability associated with hypoglycemia, the onset of which occurs while the patient is cared for in a healthcare facility												R													
			4 4 0	3 Patient death or serious physical injury associated with hypoglycemia, the onset of which occurs while the patient is being cared for in a healthcare facility		R	R						R					R					R						R
			4 4 0	4 Hypoglycemia (resulting in death or serious disability only)																									
			4 4 0	5 Onset of hypoglycemia																									
4 5 0				**HYPERBILIRUBINEMIA**																									
			4 5 0	1 Neonate hyperbilirubinemia (resulting in death or serious disability only)		2	2						2			2		2	R										2
			4 5 0	2 Death or serious disability (kernicterus) associated with failure to identify and treat hyperbilirubinemia in neonates		R	R						R						2										R

Level 1	Level 2	Level 3	Level 4	Description	NQF	JCAHO	WY	WA	UT	TX	TN	SD	SC	RI	PA	OR	NY	NJ	NV	MS	MN	ME	KS	GA-GDHR	GA-PHA	FL	CT	CO	CA
4	5	0	3	Death or serious physical injury (kernicterus) associated with failure to identify and treat hyperbilirubinimia in neonates	2										R						2						2	2	
4	5	0	4	Undiagnosed or untreated hyperbilirubinemia												R													
4	5	0	5	Patient death/harm due to failure to identify and treat hyperbilirubinimia in neonates										2	2			2			R						R		
4	6	0	0	ULCERS																									
4	6	0	1	Stage 3 or 4 ulcers acquired after admission																									
4	6	0	2	Stage 3 or 4 pressure ulcers acquired after admission to a healthcare facility	R										R	R					R							R	
4	6	0	3	Ulcers (stage 3 or 4 after admission)											R														
4	6	0	4	Venous stasis ulcer											R														
4	6	0	5	Admitted from other facility with (pressure) ulcer											R														
4	6	0	6	New (pressure) ulcer <24 hrs after admission	2										2	2		2		2	2						2		
4	6	0	7	New (pressure) ulcer >24 hrs after admission																									
4	7	0	0	SPINAL MANIPULATIVE THERAPY																									
4	7	0	1	Patient death or serious disability due to spinal manipulative therapy	R										R	R											R		
4	7	0	2	Patient death or serious physical injury due to spinal manipulative therapy											R														
4	7	0	3	Patient death/harm due to spinal manipulative therapy											R			R			R								
4	7	0	4	Complication following spinal manipulative therapy											R														
4	7	0	5	Spinal (resulting in death or serious disability only)											2	2		2		2	2						2		
4	8	0	0	SERIOUS PATIENT OUTCOMES DUE TO OTHER CARE MANAGEMENT ERRORS		2	2	2	2		2			2	2	2	2	2	2	2		2		2	2	2	2	2	
4	8	1	0	GENERAL DEATHS		2	3	2	3		3				3		3			3		3		3	3	3	2	2	
4	8	1	1	Unexpected deaths			R	R																R	R				
4	8	1	2	Any unanticipated patient death not related to the natural course of the patient's illness or underlying condition.																									

Level 1 / Level 2 / Level 3 / Level 4	Description	CA	CO	CT	FL	GA-PHA	GA-GDHR	KS	ME	MN	MS	NV	NJ	NY	OR	PA	RI	SC	SD	TN	TX	UT	WA	WY	JCAHO	NQF
	An unanticipated death unrelated to the natural course of the patient's illness or underlying condition or																									
4 8 1 3	proper treatment of that illness or underlying condition that results from the elopement of a patient who lacks the capacity to make decisions																									
4 8 1 4	Death				R				R					R						R						
4 8 1 5	Death (e.g., brain death) not directly related to natural course of patient's illness or underlying condition																									
4 8 1 6	All deaths that occur at the facility and that are directly related to any clinical service or process provided to a patient for which the patient at the time of death was not subject to "do not resuscitate" order; not in a critical care unit, except where the patient is transferred to a critical care unit as a consequence of a patient safety sentinel event that occurs elsewhere in the facility; was not in the emergency room or operating room having presented in the last 24 hours with a Glasgow score of 9 or lower		3								R	3		3		R						R				
4 8 1 7	Wrongful death																									
4 8 1 8	Other unexpected death		R											R												
4 8 2 0	DEATH OR SERIOUS OUTCOMES ATTRIBUTED TO TREATMENT PROBLEM																									
4 8 2 1	Perforations during open, laparoscopic and/or endoscopic procedures resulting in death or serious disability																									
4 8 2 2	Errors of Omission/Delay resulting in death or serious injury RELATED to the patient's underlying condition.																									
4 8 2 3	Laboratory or radiologic test results not reported to the treating practitioner or reported incorrectly which result in death or serious disability due to incorrect or missed diagnosis in the emergency department																									
4 8 2 4	Procedure Complication(s) -- Actual Death		R									R														

Level 1	Level 2	Level 3	Level 4				CA	CO	CT	FL	GA-PHA	GA-GDHR	KS	ME	MN	MS	NV	NJ	NY	OR	PA	RI	SC	SD	TN	TX	UT	WA	WY	JCAHO	NQF
			4	8	2	5 Procedure Complication(s) -- Actual Physical Injury with Permanent Loss												R														
			4	8	2	6 Procedure Complication(s) -- Actual Psychological Injury with Permanent Loss												R														
			4	8	2	7 Procedure Complication(s) -- Actual Physical and Psychological Injuries with Permanent Losses												R														
			4	8	2	8 Procedure Complication(s) -- Risk of Death												R														
			4	8	2	9 Procedure Complication(s) -- Risk of Physical Injury with Permanent Loss												R														
			4	8	2	10 Procedure Complication(s) -- Risk of Psychological Injury with Permanent Loss												R														
			4	8	2	11 Treatment Delay -- Actual Death												R														
			4	8	2	12 Treatment Delay -- Actual Physical Injury with Permanent Loss												R														
			4	8	2	13 Treatment Delay -- Actual Psychological Injury with Permanent Loss												R														
			4	8	2	14 Treatment Delay --Actual Physical and Psychological Injuries with Permanent Losses												R														
			4	8	2	15 Treatment Delay -- Risk of Death												R														
			4	8	2	16 Treatment Delay --Risk of Physical Injury with Permanent Loss												R														
			4	8	2	17 Treatment Delay -- Risk of Psychological Injury with Permanent Loss												R														
			4	8	2	18 Treatment Error -- Actual Death												R														
			4	8	2	19 Treatment Error -- Actual Physical Injury with Permanent Loss												R														
			4	8	2	20 Treatment Error -- Actual Psychological Injury with Permanent Loss												R														
			4	8	2	21 Treatment Error -- Actual Physical and Psychological Injuries with Permanent Losses												R														
			4	8	2	22 Treatment Error -- Risk of Death												R														
			4	8	2	23 Treatment Error -- Risk of Physical Injury with Permanent Loss												R														
			4	8	2	24 Treatment Error -- Risk of Psychological Injury with Permanent Loss												R														

Level 1	Level 2	Level 3	Level 4	PHYSICAL IMPAIRMENT	UT	TN	RI	NY	ME
4	8	3	0	PHYSICAL IMPAIRMENT	3	3	3	3	3
4	8	3	1	Major loss of physical or mental function that is not present when the patient is admitted to the health care facility AND is unrelated to the natural course of the patient's illness or underlying condition or proper treatment of that illness or underlying condition that results from the elopement of a patient who lacks the capacity to make decisions					
4	8	3	2	Major loss of physical or mental function not related to the natural course of the patient's illness or underlying condition	R				R
4	8	3	3	Loss of limb or organ not directly related to patient's illness or underlying condition				R	
4	8	3	4	Impairment of limb (limb unable to function at same level prior to occurrence) and impairment present at discharge or for at least 2 weeks after occurrence if patient is not discharged not resulting from patient's illness or underlying condition					
4	8	3	5	Impairment of limb (limb unable to function at same level prior to occurrence) and impairment present at discharge or for at least 2 weeks after occurrence if patient is not discharged				R	
4	8	3	6	Loss or impairment of bodily functions (sensory, motor, communication or physiologic function diminished from level prior to occurrence) and present at discharge or for at least 2 weeks after occurrence if patient is not discharged, not directly related to the natural course of the patient's illness or underlying condition		R			
4	8	3	7	Any incidence resulting in paraplegia not within normal range of patient outcomes			R	R	
4	8	3	8	Any incidence resulting in quadriplegia not within normal range of patient outcomes			R		
4	8	3	9	Any incidence resulting in any type of paralysis not within normal range of patient outcomes			R		

Level 1	Level 2	Level 3	Level 4	Description	CA	CO	CT	FL	GA-PHA	GA-GDHR	KS	ME	MN	MS	NV	NJ	NY	OR	PA	RI	SC	SD	TN	TX	UT	WA	WY	JCAHO	NQF
4	8	3	10	Any incidence resulting in impairment of sight or hearing not within normal range of patient outcomes		3		3												R			R						
4	8	3	11	Loss of limb or organ																3									
4	8	4	0	MENTAL IMPAIRMENT/BRAIN INJURY																									
4	8	4	1	Any incidence resulting in mental impairment not within normal range of patient outcomes																R									
4	8	4	2	Any incidence resulting in brain injury not within normal range of patient outcomes																									
4	8	4	3	Brain damage		R		R												R									
4	8	4	4	Brain injury as a result of occurrence involving the head AND change of consciousness level and/or loss of bodily function OR diagnostic test that shows brain injury																									
4	8	5	0	SPINAL CORD INJURY																									
4	8	5	1	Spinal damage		3		3																					
4	8	5	2	Result of an occurrence AND functional loss consistent with spinal cord injury AND permanent or temporary		R		R																					
4	8	6	0	COMBINATION OF OUTCOMES																									
4	8	6	1	Any unanticipated, usually preventable consequence of patient care that results in patient death or serious physical injury												3		3		3			3			3		3	
4	8	6	2	Incidents of unexpected death or serious injury or the risk of these that is not related to the natural course of the patient condition														R											
4	8	6	3	Any incidence resulting in loss of use of limb or organ not within normal range of patient outcomes												R				R			R						
4	8	6	4	An unanticipated death or major permanent loss of function, not related to the natural course of a patient's illness or underlying condition																						R		R	
4	8	6	5	Other event causing patient death or harm that lasts seven days or is present at discharge													3		3										
4	8	7	0	OTHER COMPLICATIONS																									
4	8	7	1	Cardiopulmonary arrest outside of ICU setting															R				3						

Level 1	Level 2	Level 3	Level 4	Description	CA	CO	CT	FL	GA-PHA	GA-GDHR	KS	ME	MN	MS	NV	NJ	NY	OR	PA	RI	SC	SD	TN	TX	UT	WA	WV	JCAHO	NQF
4	8	7	2	Cardiac and/or respiratory arrest requiring BLS/ACLS intervention not directly related to patient's illness or underlying condition													R		R				R						
4	8	7	3	Volume overload leading to pulmonary edema													R		R										
4	8	7	4	Aspiration pneumonitis/pneumonia in a non-intubated patient related to conscious sedation													R		R				R						
4	8	7	5	Catheter or tube problem																									
4	8	7	6	Other (specify)		2									2				2										
4	9	0	0	NOSOCOMIAL INFECTIONS																									
4	9	0	1	Nosocomial infections defined as reportable sentinel events by the Joint Commission on Accreditation of Healthcare Organizations (JCAHO)		R																							
4	9	0	2	Nosocomial Infection -- Actual Death											R														
4	9	0	3	Nosocomial Infection -- Actual Physical Injury with Permanent Loss											R														
4	9	0	4	Nosocomial Infection -- Actual Psychological Injury with Permanent Loss											R														
4	9	0	5	Nosocomial Infection-- Actual Physical and Psychological Injuries with Permanent Losses											R														
4	9	0	6	Nosocomial Infection -- Risk of Death											R														
4	9	0	7	Nosocomial Infection-- Risk of Physical Injury with Permanent Loss											R														
4	9	0	8	Nosocomial Infection -- Risk of Psychological Injury with Permanent Loss																									
4	9	0	9	Intravascular catheter infection															R										
4	9	0	10	Nosocomial pneumonia															R										
4	9	0	11	Sepsis 48 hrs post admit															R										
4	9	0	12	Antibiotic-associated diarrhea															R										
4	9	0	13	Antibiotic resistant organism															2										
4	10	0	0	ANESTHESIA EVENT																									
4	10	0	1	Death															R										
4	10	0	2	Cardiopulmonary arrest															R										
4	10	0	3	Myocardial infarction		2													R										

Level 1	Level 2	Level 3	Level 4		Description	CA	CO	CT	FL	GA-PHA	GA-GDHR	KS	ME	MN	MS	NV	NJ	NY	OR	PA	RI	SC	SD	TN	TX	UT	WA	WY	JCAHO	NQF
4	11	0	0																											
	4	10	0	4	Stroke		R													R										
	4	10	0	5	Occurrence as a result of anesthesia AND life-threatening complication/reaction															R										
	4	10	0	6	Use of reversal agents															R										
	4	10	0	7	Intubation trauma															R										
	4	10	0	8	Aspiration															R										
	4	10	0	9	Other (specify)															2										
					RESPIRATORY CARE																									
	4	11	0	1	Self/unplanned extubation															R										
	4	11	0	2	Unplanned/emergent intubation following a procedure/treatment/test															R										
	4	11	0	3	Ventilator alarms not set properly															R										
	4	11	0	4	Ventilator alarms inaudible															R										
	4	11	0	5	Ventilator alarms wrong/changed without authorization															R										
	4	11	0	6	Missed treatment															R										
	4	11	0	7	Other (specify)															R										
					OTHER COMPLICATIONS																									
4	12	1	0															2		2	2			2						
					EXTENDED HOSPITAL STAY/TRANSFERS																									
	4	12	1	1	Any serious or unforeseen complication, that is not expected or probable, resulting in an extended hospital stay or death of the patient													3			3										
	4	12	1	2	Hospital stay extended due to serious or unforeseen complications not within the normal range of patient outcomes													R			R										
	4	12	1	3	Patients transferred to the hospital from a diagnostic and treatment center																R										
4	12	2	0																											
					UNPLANNED PROCEDURES																									
	4	12	2	1	Any unplanned operation or reoperation (RTOR) related to the primary procedure, regardless of setting of primary procedure													3		R	3			3						
	4	12	2	2	Any unexpected operation or reoperation (RTOR) related to the primary procedure, regardless of setting of primary procedure													R		R				R						

Level 1	Level 2	Level 3	Level 4	Description	TN	RI	PA	NY
4	12		2 3	Procedure related injury requiring repair, removal of an organ, or other procedural intervention	R		3	R
4	12		2 4	Procedure related injury, requiring repair or removal of an organ				
4	12		2 5	Incorrect Procedure or Treatment - Invasive	R		R	R
4	12		2 6	Incorrect procedure or treatment that is invasive			R	
4	12		2 7	Subjecting a patient to a procedure other than that ordered or intended by the patient's attending physician			R	
4	12	3	0	EMERGENCY DEPARTMENT EVENT				
4	12		3 1	Unplanned return to ED in 48 hrs requiring admission			R	
4	12		3 2	Discrepancy between ED interpretation of X-ray or EKG and final reading		R	R	
4	12		3 3	Left without being seen			3	
4	12		3 4	Left before visit completed			R	
4	12		3 5	Other (specify)			R	
4	12	4	0	LABORATORY TEST PROBLEMS				
4	12		4 1	Test not ordered			R	
4	12		4 2	Test ordered, not performed			R	
4	12		4 3	Wrong test ordered			R	
4	12		4 4	Wrong test performed			R	
4	12		4 5	Wrong patient			R	
4	12		4 6	Wrong result			R	
4	12		4 7	Result missing or delayed			R	
4	12		4 8	Specimen quality problem			R	
4	12		4 9	Specimen delivery problem			R	
4	12		4 10	Mislabeled specimen			R	
4	12		4 11	Specimen label incomplete/missing			R	
4	12		4 12	Other (specify)			R	
4	12	5	0	OTHER			3	

Level 1	Level 2	Level 3	Level 4	Description	CA	CO	CT	FL	GA-PHA	GA-GDHR	KS	ME	MN	MS	NV	NJ	NY	OR	PA	RI	SC	SD	TN	TX	UT	WA	WV	JCAHO	NQF
4	12	5	1	IV site complication (phlebitis, bruising, infiltration)															R										
4	13	0	0	RADIOLOGY/IMAGING PROBLEMS																									
4	13	0	1	Extravasation of drug or radiologic contrast															2										
4	13	0	2	Not ordered															R										
4	13	0	3	Ordered, not performed															R										
4	13	0	4	Delay in scheduling															R										
4	13	0	5	Not completed															R										
4	13	0	6	Report unavailable/delay															R										
4	13	0	7	Incorrect reading															R										
4	13	0	8	Film unavailable or inadequate															R										
4	13	0	9	Unanticipated radiation exposure															R										
4	13	0	10	MRI safety violation															R										
4	13	0	11	Wrong procedure															R										
4	13	0	12	Wrong patient															R										
4	13	0	13	Wrong site															R										
4	13	0	14	Wrong side (L vs. R)															R										
4	13	0	15	Other (specify)															3										
4	13	1	0	REFERRAL/CONSULT PROBLEM															R										
4	13	1	1	Delay in scheduling															R										
4	13	1	2	Delay in service															R										
4	13	1	3	Report unavailable/delayed															R										
4	13	1	4	Other (specify)		2													2			2	2				2		
4	14	0	0	NEGLECT																									
4	14	0	1	Neglect or self-neglect																			R						
4	14	0	2	Any allegation of neglect																									
4	14	0	3	Neglect																									
4	14	0	4	Patient/resident neglect															I										
4	14	0	5	Neglect of an at-risk adult reportable to county department of social services OR a law-enforcement agency		R																					R		

				Description	NQF	JCAHO	WY	WA	UT	TX	TN	SD	SC	RI	PA	OR	NY	NJ	NV	MS	MN	ME	KS	GA-GDHR	GA-PHA	FL	CT	CO	CA
4	14	0	6	Any allegation of abuse or neglect of any patient or resident by any person			2					R		2	2		2		2				2						
4	14	0	7	Malnutrition or dehydration																									
				OTHER																									
4	15	0	1	Standards of care not met, with injury occurring or reasonably probable.													R						R						
4	15	0	2	Possible grounds for disciplinary action by the appropriate licensing agency.																			R						
4	15	0	3	Serious occurrence warranting DOH notification, not covered by codes 911-963.										R	R		R												
4	15	0	4	Any other incident that is reported to their malpractice insurance carrier or self-insurance program																									
4	15	0	5	Misadministration of radioactive material (as defined by BERP, Section 16.25, 10NYCRR).																									
4	15	0	6	Inappropriate discharge																									
4	15	0	7	Discharge to Wrong Family/Caregiver -- Child -- Actual Death															R										
4	15	0	8	Discharge to Wrong Family/Caregiver -- Child -- Actual Physical Injury with Permanent Loss															R										
4	15	0	9	Discharge to Wrong Family/Caregiver -- Child -- Actual Psychological Injury with Permanent Loss															R										
4	15	0	10	Discharge to Wrong Family/Caregiver -- Child -- Actual Physical and Psychological Injuries with Permanent Losses															R										
4	15	0	11	Discharge to Wrong Family/Caregiver -- Child -- Risk of Death															R										
4	15	0	12	Discharge to Wrong Family/Caregiver -- Child -- Risk of Physical Injury with Permanent Loss															R										
4	15	0	13	Discharge to Wrong Family/Caregiver -- Child -- Risk of Psychological Injury with Permanent Loss															R										
4	15	0	14	Discharge to Wrong Family/Caregiver -- Infant -- Actual Death															R										
4	15	0	15	Discharge to Wrong Family/Caregiver -- Infant -- Actual Physical Injury with Permanent Loss															R										

Level 1
Level 2   Level 3   Level 4

4   15   0   0

Level 1	Level 2	Level 3	Level 4	Description	CA	CO	CT	FL	GA-PHA	GA-GDHR	KS	ME	MN	MS	NV	NJ	NY	OR	PA	RI	SC	SD	TN	TX	UT	WA	WV	JCAHO	NQF
4	15	0	16	Discharge to Wrong Family/Caregiver -- Infant -- Actual Psychological Injury with Permanent Loss													R												
4	15	0	17	Discharge to Wrong Family/Caregiver -- Infant -- Actual Physical and Psychological Injuries with Permanent Losses													R												
4	15	0	18	Discharge to Wrong Family/Caregiver -- Infant -- Risk of Death													R												
4	15	0	19	Discharge to Wrong Family/Caregiver -- Infant -- Risk of Physical Injury with Permanent Loss													R												
4	15	0	20	Discharge to Wrong Family/Caregiver -- Infant -- Risk of Psychological Injury with Permanent Loss													R												
4	15	0	21	Discharge to Wrong Family/Caregiver -- Adult -- Actual Death													R												
4	15	0	22	Discharge to Wrong Family/Caregiver -- Adult -- Actual Physical Injury with Permanent Loss													R												
4	15	0	23	Discharge to Wrong Family/Caregiver -- Adult -- Actual Psychological Injury with Permanent Loss													R												
4	15	0	24	Discharge to Wrong Family/Caregiver -- Adult -- Actual Physical and Psychological Injuries with Permanent Losses													R												
4	15	0	25	Discharge to Wrong Family/Caregiver -- Adult -- Risk of Death													R												
4	15	0	26	Discharge to Wrong Family/Caregiver -- Adult -- Risk of Physical Injury with Permanent Loss													R												
4	15	0	27	Discharge to Wrong Family/Caregiver -- Adult -- Risk of Psychological Injury with Permanent Loss													R												
4	15	0	28	Accident																									
4	15	0	29	Accident with serious injuries																									
4	15	0	30	Other (procedure related error)															R										
4	15	0	31	Other (care management error)															R										
4	16	0	0	COMBINATION OF ABOVE					2																		R		

Level 1	Level 2	Level 3	Level 4	Event	CA	CO	CT	FL	GA-PHA	GA-GDHR	KS	ME	MN	MS	NV	NJ	NY	OR	PA	RI	SC	SD	TN	TX	UT	WA	WY	JCAHO	NQF
4	16	0	1	Care Management Event (includes death or serious disability associated with medication errors, hemolytic reaction, labor/delivery in a low risk pregnancy, hypoglycemia, kernicterus, state 3 or 4 pressure ulcers and spinal manipulative therapy)					R																					
5	0	0	0	ENVIRONMENTAL EVENTS	1																								
5	1	0	0	ELECTRIC SHOCK																									
5	1	0	1	Patient death or serious disability associated with an electric shock while being cared for in a healthcare facility		1	1		1				1		1	1	1	1	1	1	1	1			1	1		1
5	1	0	2	Electric shock (resulting in death or serious disability only)		2	2						2			2		2	2									2
5	1	0	3	Patient death or serious physical injury associated with an electric shock while being cared for in a healthcare facility																								
5	1	0	4	Electric shock to patient		R	R						R			R		R	R									R
5	1	0	5	Patient death/harm due to an electric shock																								
5	2	0	0	WRONG OR CONTAMINATED GAS/SUBSTANCES																									
5	2	0	1	Any incident in which a line designated for oxygen or other gas to be delivered to a patient contains the wrong gas or is contaminated by toxic substances		2	2						2			2		2	2		1	1						2
5	2	0	2	Any event in which a line designated for oxygen/other gas to be delivered to a patient contains the wrong gas or is contaminated by toxic substances		R	R						R			R		R	R									R
5	2	0	3	Medical gas problem																								
5	2	0	4	Wrong gas																								
5	3	0	0	SKIN INTEGRITY									R															
5	3	1	0	BURN		2	2						2			2	2	2	2				2					2
5	3	1	1	Burn (resulting in death or serious disability only)		3	3						3			3	3	3	3				3					3
5	3	1	2	Patient death or serious disability associated with a burn incurred from any source while being cared for in a healthcare facility		R	R						R															R

Level 1	Level 2	Level 3	Level 4	Description	NQF	JCAHO	WY	WA	UT	TX	TN	SD	SC	RI	PA	OR	NY	NJ	NV	MS	MN	ME	KS	GA-GDHR	GA-PHA	FL	CT	CO	CA
				Patient death or serious physical injury associated with a burn																								
5	3	1	3	incurred from any source while being cared for in a healthcare facility							R					R	R	R										R	
5	3	1	4	Patient death/harm due to a burn incurred from any source																									
5	3	1	5	Burn (electrical, chemical, thermal)																									
5	3	1	6	2nd and/or 3rd degree burns																									
5	3	1	7	Second or third degree burns AND 20% or more of body surface in an adult, or 15% or more of body surface in a child																									
5	3	2	0	OTHER											3														
5	3	2	1	Rash											R														
5	3	2	2	Abrasion											R														
5	3	2	3	Laceration											R														
5	3	2	4	Blister											R														
5	3	2	5	Other (skin integrity -- specify)	2						2				2	2	2	2	2		2							2	
5	4	0	0	FALLS	3						3					3	3	3	3		3							3	
5	4	1	0	DEATH OR OTHER INJURY																								R	
5	4	1	1	Patient death associated with a fall while being cared for in a healthcare facility	R																								
5	4	1	2	Patient death or serious physical injury associated with a fall while being cared for in a healthcare facility																									
5	4	1	3	Patient death/harm due to a fall												R		R											
5	4	1	4	Falls resulting in x-ray proven fractures, subdural or epidural hematoma, cerebral contusion, and/or internal trauma (e.g., hepatic or splenic injury)																									
5	4	1	5	Falls resulting in radiologically proven fractures, subdural or epidural hematoma, cerebral contusion, traumatic subarachnoid hemorrhage, and/or internal trauma (e.g., hepatic or splenic injury)													R				R								
5	4	1	6	Fall																									
5	4	1	7	Fall (resulting in death)							R																		

Level 1	Level 2	Level 3	Level 4		CA	CO	CT	FL	GA-PHA	GA-GDHR	KS	ME	MN	MS	NV	NJ	NY	OR	PA	RI	SC	SD	TN	TX	UT	WA	WY	JCAHO	NQF
		5 4 1	8	Fall -- Actual Death											R														
		5 4 1	9	Fall -- Actual Physical Injury with Permanent Loss											R														
		5 4 1	10	Fall -- Actual Psychological Injury with Permanent Loss											R														
		5 4 1	11	Fall -- Actual Physical and Psychological Injuries with Permanent Losses											R														
		5 4 1	12	Fall -- Risk of Death											R														
		5 4 1	13	Fall -- Risk of Physical Injury with Permanent Loss											R														
		5 4 1	14	Fall -- Risk of Psychological Injury with Permanent Loss											R														
		5 4 1	15	Falls resulting in serious disability while being cared for in a healthcare facility			R																						
5	4	2 0		ACTIVITY/LOCATION OF FALL																									
		5 4 2	1	Lying in bed															3										
		5 4 2	2	Assisted sit															R										
		5 4 2	3	Sitting at side of bed															R										
		5 4 2	4	Sitting in chair															R										
		5 4 2	5	Transferring															R										
		5 4 2	6	Ambulating															R										
		5 4 2	7	Toileting															R										
		5 4 2	8	In exam room															R										
		5 4 2	9	Hallways of facility															R										
		5 4 2	10	Grounds of facility															R										
		5 4 2	11	Other/unknown (specify)															R										
5	5	0 0		RESTRAINTS/BEDRAILS		2	2						2		2	2		2	2										2
		5 5 0	1	Restraints (resulting in death or serious disability only)																									
		5 5 0	2	Patient death or serious disability associated with the use of restraints or bedrails while being cared for in a healthcare facility									R																
		5 5 0	3	Patient death or serious physical injury associated with the use of restraints or bedrails while being cared for in a healthcare facility			R											R					2							R

Code	Level 1	Level 2	Description	CA	CO	CT	FL	GA-PHA	GA-GDHR	KS	ME	MN	MS	NV	NJ	NY	OR	PA	RI	SC	SD	TN	TX	UT	WA	WY	JCAHO	NQF
5 0 4	5	6	Patient death/harm due to the use of restraints or bedrails		R										R													
5 0 5	5	6	Death resulting from restraint															R				R						
5 0 6	5	6	Death or injury in restraints																									
5 0 7	5	6	Restraint related incident											R														
5 0 8	5	6	Restraint -- Actual Death											R														
5 0 9	5	6	Restraint -- Actual Physical Injury with Permanent Loss											R														
5 0 10	5	6	Restraint -- Actual Psychological Injury with Permanent Loss																									
5 0 11	5	6	Restraint -- Actual Physical and Psychological Injuries with Permanent Losses											R														
5 0 12	5	6	Restraint -- Risk of Death											R														
5 0 13	5	6	Restraint -- Risk of Physical Injury with Permanent Loss											R														
5 0 14	5	6	Restraint -- Risk of Psychological Injury with Permanent Loss																									
5 6 1 0	5	6	SERVICE DISRUPTION DUE TO ADVERSE CONDITIONS OR DISASTER													2		2	2		2	2			2			
5 6 1 1	5	6	Service disruption due to adverse manmade conditions or disaster															3										
5 6 1 2	5	6	Service disruption due to adverse natural conditions or disaster															1										
5 6 2 0	5	6	TERMINATION OF SERVICES. Unscheduled termination of any services vital to the continued safe operation of the hospital or to the health and safety of its patients and personnel													3		1	3			3						
5 6 2 1	5	6	safe operation of the hospital or to the health and safety of its patients and personnel. Termination of any services vital to the continued safe operation of the hospital or to the health and safety of its patients and personnel, including but not																									
5 6 2 2	5	6	limited to the anticipated or actual termination of telephone, electric, gas, fuel, water, heat, air conditioning, rodent or pest control, laundry services, food or contract services													R			R									

Level 1	Level 2	Level 3	Level 4	Description	CA	CO	CT	FL	GA-PHA	GA-GDHR	KS	ME	MN	MS	NV	NJ	NY	OR	PA	RI	SC	SD	TN	TX	UT	WA	WY	JCAHO	NQF
5	6		2	Termination of any services vital to the continued safe operation of the facility or to the health and safety of its patients and personnel, including but not limited to the anticipated or actual termination of telephone, electric, gas, fuel, water, heat, air conditioning, rodent or pest control, laundry services, food or contract services															3			3	R			3			
5	6	3	0	INTERRUPTION OF SERVICES																									
5	6	3	1	Interruption or termination of any clinical service															I										
5	6	3	2	Interruption of utility service															I										
5	6	3	3	Loss of utilities, such as electricity, natural gas, telephone, emergency generator, fire alarm, sprinklers, and other critical equipment necessary for operation of the facility for more than 24 hrs																									
5	6	3	4	A failure or major malfunction of a facility system such as the heating, ventilation, fire alarm, fire sprinkler, electrical, electronic information management, or water supply which affects any patient diagnosis, treatment, or care service within the facility															3			R				R			
5	6	4	0	OTHER																									
5	6	4	1	Other (infrastructure failure)															I	2							2		
5	7	0	0	INFECTIOUS OUTBREAKS	2															R							R		
5	7	0	1	Infectious outbreaks																									
5	7	0	2	Infection outbreaks as defined by the department in regulation																									
5	7	0	3	Infection control																									
5	7	0	4	Epidemic outbreaks	R																								
5	7	0	5	Prevalence of communicable disease	R																								
5	8	0	0	STRIKES													2		2	2			2						
5	8	0	1	Strike by hospital staff													R			R			R						
5	8	0	2	Strike by facility staff																									
5	8	0	3	Strikes by personnel																									

Level 1	Level 2	Level 3	Level 4	Description	CA	CO	CT	FL	GA-PHA	GA-GDHR	KS	ME	MN	MS	NV	NJ	NY	OR	PA	RI	SC	SD	TN	TX	UT	WA	WV	JCAHO	NQF
5	8	0	4	Pending strike	2												2		I	2		2	2						
5	8	0	5	Receipt of strike notice																R									
5	9	0	0	EMERGENCY SITUATIONS/DISASTERS																									
5	9	0	1	Disasters or other emergency situations external to the hospital environment which adversely affect facility operations															I										
5	9	0	2	External disaster outside the control of the hospital which affects facility operations													R		I				R						
5	9	0	3	External disaster outside the control of the facility which affects facility operations															I										
5	9	0	4	Emergency services																									
5	9	0	5	Hospital in divert status																									
5	9	0	6	EMTALA violation																									
5	9	0	7	Activation of internal or external emergency plan																									
5	9	0	8	Partial or complete evacuation of the facility resulting from natural disaster																		R							
5	9	0	9	Other catastrophes and unusual occurrences that threaten the welfare, safety, or health of patients, personnel, or visitors	R																								
5	10	0	0	POISONING	2												2			2			2						
5	10	0	1	Poisoning occurring within the hospital (water, air, food)													R			R			R						
5	10	0	2	Poisoning occurring within the facility (water, air, food or ingestion)																									
5	10	0	3	Poisoning involving patients in the facility																									
5	10	0	4	Poisoning	R																								
5	11	0	0	FIRE																									
5	11	0	1	Fire	2												2			2	2	2	2			2			
5	11	0	2	A fire which affects any patient diagnosis, treatment, or care area of the facility	R																2	2				R			
5	11	0	3	Any fire with structural damage or where injury or death occurs																									
5	11	0	4	Hospital fire disrupting patient care or causing harm to patients or staff													R					R							

Level 1	Level 2	Level 3	Level 4	Description	CA	CO	CT	FL	GA-PHA	GA-GDHR	KS	ME	MN	MS	NV	NJ	NY	OR	PA	RI	SC	SD	TN	TX	UT	WA	WY	JCAHO	NQF
5	11	0	5	Facility fire disrupting patient care or causing harm to patients or staff																			R						
5	11	0	6	All other fires (not those disrupting patient care or causing harm to patients and staff)																			R						
5	11	0	7	Fires or internal disasters in the facility which disrupt the provisions of patient care services or cause harm to patients or personnel																									
5	11	0	8	Anticipated closure or discontinuation of service at least 30 days in advance																									
5	11	0	9	Every fire regardless of size or damage that occurs in the facility																R									
5	12	0	0	ADMINISTRATION AND MANAGEMENT PROBLEMS																									
5	12	0	1	Error in patient billing/records															2			R							
5	12	0	2	Missing or incorrect patient ID															1										
5	12	0	3	Incomplete/incorrect order entry information															1										
5	12	0	4	Failure to report Health Department reportable diseases															1										
5	12	0	5	Narcotics discrepancy					2										1		R								
5	13	0	0	COMBINATION OF ABOVE																									
5	13	0	1	Environmental event (includes death or serious disability associated with electric shock, contaminated gas line, burns, falls, and restraints/bedrails)					R										1										
5	14	0	0	OTHER	2								2		2	2					2		2						
5	14	0	1	Other event causing patient death or harm that lasts seven days or is present at discharge												R													
5	14	0	2	Other -- Actual Death											R														
5	14	0	3	Other -- Actual Physical Injury with Permanent Loss											R														
5	14	0	4	Other -- Actual Psychological Injury with Permanent Loss											R														
5	14	0	5	Other -- Actual Physical and Psychological Injuries with Permanent Losses											R														
5	14	0	6	Other -- Risk of Death											R														

Level 1	Level 2	Level 3	Level 4	Description	CA	CO	CT	FL	GA-PHA	GA-GDHR	KS	ME	MN	MS	NV	NJ	NY	OR	PA	RI	SC	SD	TN	TX	UT	WA	WY	JCAHO	NQF
5	14	0	7	Other -- Risk of Physical Injury with Permanent Loss											R														
5	14	0	8	Other -- Risk of Psychological Injury with Permanent Loss											R														
5	14	0	9	Accidents or incidents occurring in the facility, including medication errors and adverse drug reactions, which involve patients, staff, or visitors that result in death or serious injuries or hospitalization	R								R								R								
5	14	0	10	Major accidents																									
5	14	0	11	Not one of the (NQF) 27																			R						
5	14	0	12	All other unusual incidents or accident warranting DOH notification, not covered by codes																									
5	14	0	13	Infestation by parasites or vectors	R																								
6	0	0	0	**CRIMINAL EVENTS**	1	1	1		1	1		1	1	1	1		1		1			1	1	1	1	1	1	1	1
6	1	0	0	IMPERSONATION OF HEALTH CARE PROVIDER																									
6	1	0	1	Criminal event (includes any instance of impersonating a healthcare provider, patient abduction, sexual assault and death or serious disability from physical assault)			2		2				2						2									2	2
6	1	0	2	Any instance of care ordered by or provided by someone impersonating a physician, nurse, pharmacist, or other licensed healthcare provider																									
6	1	0	3	Care ordered/provided by one impersonating a licensed healthcare worker			R		R				R		R				1				R						R
6	1	0	4	Impersonation																									
6	2	0	0	PATIENT ABDUCTION																									
6	2	0	1	Abduction of a patient of any age			2						2		2		2		2				2	2	2	2	2	2	2
6	2	0	2	Abduction		R							R																
6	2	0	3	Patient abduction																									
6	2	0	4	Adult abduction																									
6	2	0	5	Abduction -- Adult -- Actual Death											R								R		R				
6	2	0	6	Abduction -- Adult -- Actual Physical Injury with Permanent Loss											R														

Level 1	Level 2	Level 3	Level 4	Description	CA	CO	CT	FL	GA-PHA	GA-GDHR	KS	ME	MN	MS	NV	NJ	NY	OR	PA	RI	SC	SD	TN	TX	UT	WA	WY	JCAHO	NQF
6	2	0	7	Abduction -- Adult -- Actual Psychological Injury with Permanent Loss											R														
6	2	0	8	Abduction -- Adult -- Actual Physical and Psychological Injuries with Permanent Losses											R				I										
6	2	0	9	Abduction -- Adult -- Risk of Death											R														
6	2	0	10	Abduction -- Adult -- Risk of Physical Injury with Permanent Loss											R														
6	2	0	11	Abduction -- Adult -- Risk of Psychological Injury with Permanent Loss											R														
6	2	0	12	Disappearance of infant from nursery																			R						
6	2	0	13	The abduction of a newborn infant patient from the hospital or the discharge of a newborn infant patient from the hospital into the custody of an individual in circumstances in which the hospital knew, or in the exercise of ordinary care should have known, that the individual did not have legal custody of the infant													R		I					R					
6	2	0	14	Disappearance of child from pediatrics																									
6	2	0	15	Infant Abduction											R														
6	2	0	16	Abduction -- Infant -- Actual Death											R														
6	2	0	17	Abduction -- Infant -- Actual Physical Injury with Permanent Loss											R														
6	2	0	18	Abduction -- Infant -- Actual Psychological Injury with Permanent Loss											R														
6	2	0	19	Abduction -- Infant -- Actual Physical and Psychological Injuries with Permanent Losses											R														
6	2	0	20	Abduction -- Infant -- Risk of Death											R														
6	2	0	21	Abduction -- Infant -- Risk of Physical Injury with Permanent Loss											R														
6	2	0	22	Abduction -- Infant -- Risk of Psychological Injury with Permanent Loss											R														
6	2	0	23	Abduction -- Child -- Actual Death											R														
6	2	0	24	Abduction -- Child -- Actual Physical Injury with Permanent Loss											R														

Level 1	Level 2	Level 3	Level 4	Item	CA	CO	CT	FL	GA-PHA	GA-GDHR	KS	ME	MN	MS	NV	NJ	NY	OR	PA	RI	SC	SD	TN	TX	UT	WA	WY	JCAHO	NQF
6	2	0	25	Abduction -- Child -- Actual Psychological Injury with Permanent Loss													R												
6	2	0	26	Abduction -- Child -- Actual Physical and Psychological Injuries with Permanent Losses													R												
6	2	0	27	Abduction -- Child -- Risk of Death													R												
6	2	0	28	Abduction -- Child -- Risk of Physical Injury with Permanent Loss													R												
6	2	0	29	Abduction -- Child -- Risk of Psychological Injury with Permanent Loss													R												
6	2	0	30	Infant abduction or discharge to the wrong family																									
6	2	0	31	An infant abduction or discharge to the wrong family																									
6	3	0		SEXUAL ASSAULT		2	2		2	2		2	2		2		2		2				2	2	2	2		2	2
6	3	0	1	Sexual assault on a patient within or on the grounds of a healthcare facility			R					R	R												R	R		R	R
6	3	0	2	Sexual assault																									
6	3	0	3	Rape of a patient																									
6	3	0	4	Rape of a patient (includes alleged rape with clinical confirmation)											R														
6	3	0	5	Rape													R												
6	3	0	6	Rape -- Actual Death													R												
6	3	0	7	Rape -- Actual Physical Injury with Permanent Loss													R												
6	3	0	8	Rape -- Actual Psychological Injury with Permanent Loss																									
6	3	0	9	Rape -- Actual Physical and Psychological Injuries with Permanent Losses													R												
6	3	0	10	Rape -- Risk of Death													R												
6	3	0	11	Rape -- Risk of Physical Injury with Permanent Loss													R												
6	3	0	12	Rape -- Risk of Psychological Injury with Permanent Loss													R												
6	3	0	13	Any rape of a patient which occurs in the hospital					R																				
6	3	0	14	Rape by another patient or staff						R													R						
6	3	0	15	Resident to resident altercations																			R						

Level 1	Level 2	Level 3	Level 4	Description	CA	CO	CT	FL	GA-PHA	GA-GDHR	KS	MR	MN	MS	NV	NJ	NY	OR	PA	RI	SC	SD	TN	TX	UT	WA	WY	JCAHO	NQF
6	3	0	16	The sexual assault of a patient during treatment or while the patient was on the premises of the hospital or facility	R	R													I				R	R		R			
6	3	0	17	Sexual assault or rape of a patient or staff member while in the hospital																									
6	3	0	18	Sexual assault/rape																									
6	3	0	19	Sexual abuse																									
6	3	0	20	Sexual abuse committed knowingly AND consent not given AND sexual intrusion, or penetration, or touching intimate body parts or the clothing covering intimate body parts, or examining, or treating clients for other than bona fide medical purposes, or observing or photographing client's intimate parts, or physical force/threat																									
6	3	0	21	Sexual acts involving patients who are minors, nonconsenting adults, or persons incapable of consent																									
6	4	0	0	PHYSICAL ASSAULT	2	2	2						2		2	2	2		2			2	2		2				2
6	4	0	1	Death or significant injury of a patient or staff member resulting from a physical assault (i.e., battery) that occurs within or on the grounds of a healthcare facility		R							R																
6	4	0	2	Physical assault (resulting in death or significant injury only)																									
6	4	0	3	Death resulting from other than natural causes originating on facility property such as accidents, abuse, negligence, or suicide																									
6	4	0	4	Intentional injury to a patient, whether by staff or others	R	R																R	R		R				
6	4	0	5	Physical abuse																									
6	4	0	6	Physical abuse with intent AND bodily injury and/or serious bodily injury, and/or unreasonable confinement or restraint																									
6	4	0	7	Assault by staff															I										
6	4	0	8	Assault by patient															I										
6	4	0	9	Assault by visitor															I										

Level 1	Level 2	Level 3	Level 4	Description	CA	CO	CT	FL	GA-PHA	GA-GDHR	KS	ME	MN	MS	NV	NJ	NY	OR	PA	RI	SC	SD	TN	TX	UT	WA	WY	JCAHO	NQF
6	4	0	10	Physical assaults on inmate-patients, employees, or visitors	R																								
6	4	0	11	Criminal act																									
6	4	0	12	Homicide -- Actual Death											R														
6	4	0	13	Homicide -- Actual Physical Injury with Permanent Loss											R														
6	4	0	14	Homicide -- Actual Psychological Injury with Permanent Loss											R														
6	4	0	15	Homicide -- Psychological Injuries with Permanent Losses											R														
6	4	0	16	Homicide -- Risk of Death											R														
6	4	0	17	Homicide -- Risk of Physical Injury with Permanent Loss											R		R						R						
6	4	0	18	Homicide -- Risk of Psychological Injury with Permanent Loss											R														
6	4	0	19	Crime resulting in death or serious injury																									
6	4	0	20	Crime resulting in death or serious injury to a patient																									
6	4	0	21	Assault -- Actual Death											R														
6	4	0	22	Assault -- Actual Physical Injury with Permanent Loss											R														
6	4	0	23	Assault -- Actual Psychological Injury with Permanent Loss											R														
6	4	0	24	Assault -- Actual Physical and Psychological Injuries with Permanent Losses											R														
6	4	0	25	Assault -- Risk of Death											R														
6	4	0	26	Assault -- Risk of Physical Injury with Permanent Loss											R														
6	4	0	27	Assault -- Risk of Psychological Injury with Permanent Loss											R														
6	5	0	0	VERBAL OR UNSPECIFIED ASSAULT		2								2	R				2				2				2		
6	5	0	1	Verbal abuse															1										
6	5	0	2	Verbal abuse committed knowingly and a threat OR physical action (including threatening gesture) and fear																									
6	5	0	3	Abuse		R								R									R				R		
6	5	0	4	Any allegation of abuse																									

Level 1	Level 2	Level 3	Level 4		CA	CO	CT	FL	GA-PHA	GA-GDHR	KS	MR	MN	MS	NV	NJ	NY	OR	PA	RI	SC	SD	TN	TX	UT	WA	WY	JCAHO	NQF
6	6	0	0	SUSPICIOUS DEATH OR INJURY	2	2								2													2		
6	6	0	1	Injury of unknown origin																									
6	6	0	2	Unexplained injuries or bruises	R	R								R													R		
6	6	0	3	Occurrence resulting in death and reportable to the coroner as unexplained or suspicious																									
6	6	0	4	Death from unnatural causes																									
6	7	0	0	MISAPPROPRIATION	2	2													2				2				2		
6	7	0	1	Misappropriation																									
6	7	0	2	Misappropriation of resident/patient/client property																									
6	7	0	3	Deliberate misplacing, exploiting, or wrongful use of client's property OR pattern of misplacing, exploiting, or wrongful use of a client's property AND client consent not given	R	R																	R				R		
6	7	0	4	Misappropriation of funds																									
6	7	0	5	Diverted drugs -- deliberate																									
6	7	0	6	Drug diversion/theft															1										
6	7	0	7	Misappropriation of patient/resident property		R													1										
6	8	0	0	OTHER POTENTIALLY CRIMINAL ACTIVITIES	2														2										
6	8	0	1	Threat by patient															1										
6	8	0	2	Confrontational behavior															1										
6	8	0	3	Consensual sexual activity															1										
6	8	0	4	Other potentially criminal activities															1										
6	8	0	5	Other occurrence (Describe)																									
6	8	0	6	All suspected criminal activity involving inmate-patients, employees, or visitors	R																								

REFERENCES

Bagian, J.P., C. Lee, J. Gosbee, J. DeRosier, E. Stalhandske, N. Eldridge, R. Williams, and M. Burkhardt. "Developing and Deploying a Patient Safety Program in a Large Health Care Delivery System: You Can't Fix What You Don't Know About," *Joint Communication Journal of Quality Improvement*, 2000, 27, 522-532.

Battles, J.B., H.S. Kaplan, T.W. Van der Schaff, and C.E. Shea. "The Attributes of Medical Event Reporting Systems: Experience with a Prototype Medical Event Reporting System for Transfusion Medicine," *Archives of Pathology and Laboratory Medicine*, 1998, 122, 231-238.

Cohen, M.R. "Why Error Reporting Systems Should Be Voluntary: They Provide Better Information for Reducing Errors," *British Medical Journal*, 2000, 320, 728-729.

Department of Veterans Affairs. *National Center for Patient Safety Triage Cards for Root Cause Analysis*, Ann Arbor, MI: Veterans Health Administration, 2001.

Farley, D., S.C. Morton, C. Damberg, A.M. Fremont, S.H. Berry, M.D. Greenberg, et al. *Assessment of the National Patient Safety Initiative: Context and Baseline Evaluation Report 1*, Santa Monica, CA: RAND, TR-203-AHRQ, 2005.

Flowers, L. and T. Riley. *How States Are Responding to Medical Errors: An Analysis of Recent State Legislative Proposals*, Portland, ME: National Academy for State Health Policy, 2000.

Flowers, L. and T. Riley. *State-Based Mandatory Reporting of Medical Errors: An Analysis of Legal and Policy Issues*, Portland, ME: National Academy for State Health Policy, 2001.

Gaul, G. M. "Plan Would Compile, Analyze Medical Errors: Measure Awaits Bush's Signature Encourages Confidential Reporting to Improve Health Care, *Washington Post*, July 29, 2005, A.06.

Institute of Medicine. *To Err is Human: Building a Safer Health System*, Washington, DC: National Academy Press, 2000.

Institute of Medicine. *Patient Safety: Achieving a New Standard for Care*, Washington, DC: National Academy Press, 2004.

IOM—*See* Institute of Medicine.

Kaplan, H.L. MERS-TM: Medical Event Reporting System for Transfusion Medicine: Reference Manual, Version 3.0, New York, NY: Trustees of Colombia University, 2001.

Kraman, S.S. & G. Hamm. "Risk Management: Extreme Honesty May Be the Best Policy," *Annals of Internal Medicine,* 1999, 131, (12), 963-967.

Leape, L. "Reporting of Adverse Events," *New England Journal of Medicine*, 2002, 347 (20), 1633-1638.

McGlynn, E.A., S.M. Asch, J. Adams, J. Keesey, J. Hicks, A. DeCristofaro, and E.A. Kerr. "The Quality of Health Care Delivered to Adults in the United States," *New England Journal of Medicine*, June 26 2003, 348 (26), 2635-2264.

National Quality Forum. *Serious Reportable Events in Healthcare*, Washington, DC: National Forum for Health Care Quality Measurement and Reporting, 2002.

New York State Department of Health, "NYPORTS-The New York Patient Occurrence and Tracking System-Annual Report 1999," 2001, www.health.state.ny.us/press/releases/2001/nyports/nyports.htm#intro.

NQF—*See* National Quality Forum.

Tang, P. Public Briefing on IOM Patient Safety: Achieving a New Standard for Care (http://www4.nationalacademies.org/news.nsf/isbn/s0309090776?OpenDocument), 2003.

Riley, T. *Improving Patient Safety: What States Can Do About Medical Errors,* Portland, ME: National Academy of State Health Policy, 2000.

Rosenthal, J. and T. Riley. *Patient Safety and Medical Errors: A Road Map for State Action*, Portland, ME: National Academy for State Health Policy, 2001.

Rosenthal, J., T. Riley, and M. Booth. *Medical Errors and Adverse Events: A Report of a 50-State Survey*, Portland: ME, National Academy for State Health Policy, 2000.

Rosenthal, J., M. Booth, L. Flowers, & T. Riley. *Current State Programs Addressing Medical Errors: An Analysis of Medical Reporting and Other Initiatives*, Portland, ME: National Academy of State Health Policy, 2001.

Rosenthal, J. & M. Booth. *Defining Reportable Adverse Events: A Guide for States Tracking Medical Errors,* Portland, ME: National Academy for State Health Policy, 2003.

Rozich, J.D., C.R. Haraden, and R.K. Resar. "Adverse Drug Event Trigger Tool: A Practical Methodology for Measuring Medication

Related Harm." *Quality and Safety in Health Care*, 12, 2003, 194-200.

Scott, H.D., S E. Rosenbaum, W.J. Waters, A.M. Colt, L.G. Andrews, J.P. Juergens, et al. "Rhode Island Physicians' Recognition and Reporting of Adverse Drug Reactions." *Rhode Island Medical Journal*, 1987, 70, 311-316.

Strom, B.L. and P. Tugwell. "Pharmacoepidemiology: Current Status, Prospects, and Problems." *Annals of Internal Medicine*, 1990, 113, 179-181.

U.S. Pharmacopeia. *Summary of Information Submitted to MedMARx in the Year 2002: The Quest for Quality*, Rockville. MD: The United States Pharmacopeial Convention, Inc., 2003.